Survival Kit for MRCP Part 2

We dedicate this book to our parents and to the following eminent teachers and physicians:

B. M. Hegde, S. Dwiwedi, G. N. Kundaje, P. Shatapathy, Dato I. Merican, C. Oakley, J. Calam, A. Owen, D. Lythall, I. Sturgess, P. Nihoyanopoulos, H. Hodgson, I. Palacious, D. J. M. Sinclair, N. Rowell, M. A. de Belder, A. Davies, J. Hall, D. N. Bateman, A. Ashraf, A. Kenny, R Bexton, D. Reid, J. McCoomb, J. Cleland, P. Bourdillon, Dato-Seri Mahatir Mohamad, S. Easaw, P. Kaur, J. Cash, K. A. Abraham, Z. Kasih, Y. S. Rai, J. P. Bourke, S. Kingston, P. D. Higham, S. Motwani and Dato Jai Mohan

Survival Kit
for
MRCP Part 2

W. M. Chong
Associate College Tutor, Royal College of Physicians (London)
and
Registrar in Cardiology, Department of Cardiology
Regional Cardiac Centre, South Cleveland Hospital
Cleveland, UK

K. C. Wong
Registrar in Medicine, Department of Medicine
Regional Cardiac Centre, South Cleveland Hospital
Cleveland, UK

with Forewords by

Professor John Calam
Professor of Gastroenterology
Department of Medicine
Royal Postgraduate Medical School
Hammersmith Hospital
University of London, UK

Professor Philip Samet
The First Chief of Staff and Professor of Cardiology
Department of Cardiology
Mount Sinai Medical Center
University of Miami, USA

Dr A. Das
Senior Staff Cardiac Surgeon
Department of Cardiac Surgery
University Medical Centre
Kasturba Medical College
India

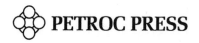 PETROC PRESS

Petroc Press, an imprint of LibraPharm Limited

Distributors

Plymbridge Distributors Limited, Plymbridge House, Estover Road, Plymouth PL6 7PZ, UK

Published 1998 by LibraPharm Limited, 3 Thames Court, High Street, Goring-on-Thames, Reading, Berks RG8 9AR, UK

A catalogue record for this book is available from the British Library

ISBN 1 900603 06 3

Typeset by Richard Powell Editorial and Production Services, Basingstoke, Hampshire RG22 4TX

Printed and bound in Great Britain by
Redwood Books, Trowbridge, Wiltshire BA14 8RN

Contents

Foreword

It is a pleasure and privilege to write a foreword for this excellent collection of clinical questions and answers. Dr Chong and Dr Wong, who have been my colleagues at the Hammersmith Hospital, have dedicated their extensive clinical experience into case-solving problem based learning. They pose relevant questions and provide answers that would satisfy the examiners. The cases are drawn from all of the medical sub-specialities of internal medicine and the material is presented in a lively and instructive format.

This book will be invaluable to anyone wishing to refresh their knowledge of internal medicine, but particularly essential to those revising for the MRCP Part 2, because these are exactly the sort of cases in which candidates will have to excel in this examination. The approach to solving the cases reflects the use of thought processes: heuristics, causal reasoning and lateral thinking, which will help the reader to become a more effective physician and to pass the examination!

London, 1997

Professor John Calam, MD, FRCP
Professor of Medicine
Department of Medicine
Royal Postgraduate Medical School
Hammersmith Hospital
University of London
UK

Foreword

In this book Dr Wong and Dr Chong clearly reflect the clinical approaches, so well championed in British medicine, of the solution of patient problems. Many American cardiologists, and I include myself in this category, who trained in the 1950s and 1960s in the combined use of clinical and physiological data, have witnessed with concern a perceived decrease in the emphasis on the utilisation of clinical skills by some of our colleagues.

In cardiology, for example, over-reliance on technology cannot always replace skills such as history taking, physical examination, classic electrocardiography, fluoroscopy and roentgenology. There is the very real danger that we will lose the art of medicine so well typified by Osler.

The methodology that this Survival Kit teaches emphasises the use of heuristics and lateral thinking and these two talented cardiologists are to be congratulated on producing a text that will be valuable to all physicians, and especially cardiologists, in training and as preparation for their professional examinations.

Miami, 1997

Dr Philip Samet, MD, FACC
The First Chief of Staff and Professor of Cardiology
Department of Cardiology
Mount Sinai Medical Centre
University of Miami
USA

Foreword

It is both a pleasure and a privilege to write this foreword to these two dedicated cardiologists' book. The book itself is an exceptionally useful tool for any sincere undergraduate or postgraduate student of the art and craft of cardiology. As Hypocrites said, 'Life is short but art is long'. May this book make the transition from physician to cardiologist a less painful one.

Drs Chong (Chief of Cardiology, Consultant Cardiologist) and Wong (Senior Registrar in Cardiology) have pioneered an intervention cardiological academic unit at the University Medical Centre of Kasturba College. Together we have shared the development of interventional cardiology, which began with Andreas Gruentzig's PTCA and the quantum development of stent deployment and the percutaneous transmitral commissurotomy utilising a metallic dilator.

Interventional cardiology is an art and craft with few experts and little room for error. My hope is that this book will help those in search of excellence. As a fellow cardiologist, I share their dreams, aspirations and compassion, and hope that this book will be a useful tool for those who seek the necessary knowledge. I wish all who read it a successful career.

Kasturba, 1998

A. Das, MS, MCh(JIPMER)
Senior Staff Cardiac Surgeon
Department of Cardiac Surgery
University Medical Centre
Kasturba Medical College

Preface

By reading this page, you are searching for a solution. What is the best book for the MRCP, MMed(Int Med), FCP(SA), FRACP, FRCP(C) or the Diploma of Internal Medicine of the American Boards? There is no such book, since we have evolved intellectually to have different needs. The PET scan reveals that some think visually and others in words. In the era of the MMX chip and the interactive CD-ROM, visual data is accessible by the megabyte, which is why we have not provided a token series of pictures. All of these elite examinations are linked by a need to demonstrate the possession of certain criteria. Among them are compassion, the ability fluently to elicit clinical signs under pressure and the capacity to abstract information under stress. The diagnostic process involves the dynamic interplay of data acquisition (visual, numerical or tactile), thinking and knowledge, which may be likened to the dance of Shiva (named after the nuclear reactor and the Hindu God of destruction which precedes creation). These are not a menagerie of questions and answers but an illustration of the use of heuristics, lateral thinking, causal reasoning, pathophysiological reasoning, diagnostic verification and the demonstration of possible pitfalls, errors in thought and an expansion of the subtle variation in details which makes the critical difference. As the distinguished physician and MRCP examiner, Professor H. de Wardener FRCP said, 'As regards diagnosis, I am more interested in his thinking. If his thinking is all right, he is all right', thus the need for this book.

The term *survival* is aptly chosen, as a famous strategist, Sun Tzu said, 'One can never prepare to win a battle, but one can always ensure that one is not defeated.' It is a truism in life that all things change (for example, with the advent of molecular biology), and this book provides the cognitive tools for adaptation. Science will advance but the methodology will remain unchanged. For example, Hippocrates of Cos described the relationship between galactorrhoea in pregnancy and miscarriage, long before we understood the inhibitory role of dopamine in the release of prolactin. Luck is the point where preparation and determination meet opportunity, and the lessons learned will make the difference between a house painter and Michaelangelo. We also take this opportunity to wish you the best of luck in your examination, and a successful career.

Hammersmith, London, 1998   WMC
                                                                               KCW

Acknowledgements

We are grateful for the editorial advice of **Dr Hui Ying Ming**, BSc, MBBS, of the Hammersmith Hospital, London, and **Miss Hui Chi Ming**, UMDS Guys and St Thomas' Medical School. **Miss Terrie Yap**, BSc, UKM, has kindly acted as our marketing adviser. We also express our sincere gratitude to **Dr Peter Clarke** and **Mr Richard Powell** of LibraPharm Limited for their unflinching support, advice and patience during the design, editorial, production and marketing stages of this project.

The following eminent consultants reviewed appropriate sections of this book. We are grateful for their comments and advice, but we accept responsibility for any errors or omissions.

Cardiology

Dr Philip Samet, MD, FACC, Professor of Cardiology, Mount Sinai Medical Center, University of Miami School of Medicine, USA.

Dr A. Tolentino, MD, FACC, Consultant Cardiologist, Mount Sinai Medical Center, University of Miami School of Medicine, USA.

Dr Gerald Maurer, MD, FACC, Professor of Cardiology, Chairman and Head, Department of Cardiology, AKH University Hospital, University of Vienna, Austria.

Respiratory Medicine

Dr L. H. Block, MD, Professor of Pulmonology, Chairman and Head, Department of Pulmonology, AKH University Hospital, University of Vienna, Austria.

Dr Tahir Ahmed, MD, FACP, FCCP, Professor of Medicine, Mount Sinai Medical Center, Chief of Respiratory Medicine. University of Miami School of Medicine, USA.

Gastroenterology

Dr Jamie Barkin, MD, FACP, Master of the American College of Gastroenterology; Governor of the American College of Physicians; Professor of Medicine, Chief of Gastroenterology, Mount Sinai Medical Center, University of Miami School of Medicine, USA.

Dr John Calam, MA, MD, FRCP, Professor of Gastroenterology, Division of Gastroenterology and Consultant Gastroenterologist, Royal Postgraduate Medical School, Hammersmith Hospital, University of London, UK.

Emergency Medicine

Dr **Arthur Diskin**, MD, FACEP, Chairman of the Department of Emergency Medicine and Examiner for the American Boards of Emergency Medicine, Mount Sinai Medical Center, University of Miami School of Medicine, USA.

Dr **Michael Zimpfer**, MD, Chairman of the Department of Anaesthesiology, Intensive Care and Emergency Medicine, and Professor of Medicine, AKH University Hospital, University of Vienna, Austria.

Dr **Claudia Müller**, MD, Associate Professor of the Department of Anaesthesiology, Intensive Care and Emergency Medicine, AKH University Hospital, University of Vienna, Austria.

Haematology

Dr **J. Byrnes**, MD, FACP, Chief of Hematology and Oncology, Director of the William J. Harrington Center for Blood Diseases, Jackson Memorial Hospital, Professor of Medicine, University of Miami School of Medicine, USA.

Dr **Daniel Nixon**, MD, FACP, Director of the Comprehensive Cancer Center, Department of Hematology and Oncology, Mount Sinai Medical Center, University of Miami School of Medicine, USA.

Endocrinology and Metabolic Medicine

Dr **Morton J. Robinson**, MD, Chairman, Department of Pathology and Metabolic Medicine, Professor of Pathology and Metabolic Medicine, Mount Sinai Medical Center, University of Miami School of Medicine, USA.

Dr **W. Waldhausl**, MD, Chairman, Department of Endocrinology and Metabolic Medicine, Professor of Medicine, AKH University Hospital, University of Vienna, Austria.

Nephrology

Dr **Walter H. Hörl**, MD, Chairman, Department of Nephrology and Dialysis, Professor of Medicine, AKH University Hospital, University of Vienna, Austria.

Dr **Leticia Adan**, MD, Medical Director, Department of Nephrology, Mount Sinai Medical Center, University of Miami School of Medicine, USA

Neurology

Dr **Luder Deecke**, MD, Chairman, Department of Clinical Neurology, Professor of Neurology, AKH University Hospital, University of Vienna, Austria.

Dr Edward Auff, MD, Chairman, Department of Rehabilitation Neurology, Professor of Medicine, AKH University Hospital, University of Vienna, Austria.

Infectious Diseases

Dr Wolfgang Graninger, MD, Head of the Department of Infectious Diseases, Professor of Infectious Diseases and Internal Medicine, AKH University Hospital, University of Vienna, Austria.

Dr Joseph Chan, MD, FACP, Associate Professor of Medicine, Division of Infectious diseases and Travel Medicine, Mount Sinai Medical Center, University of Miami School of Medicine, USA.

General Medicine

Dr Gloria Weinberg, MD, FACP, Chief of Ambulatory Medicine, Director of the Internal Medicine Residency, Mount Sinai Medical Center, University of Miami School of Medicine, USA.

Dr Conrad Fischer, MD, Consultant Physician in Internal Medicine, Director of Training Program for Medicine for the National Boards in Medical Sciences Bellevue Hospital, New York University, New York, USA.

IT Medicine

Mr Michael Chong, MSc, Systems Consultant, has designed mathematical models of non-linear diagnostic reasoning to analyse the questions. This has elucidated the role of heuristics alongside classic approaches to medicine.

This text was reviewed by several physicians preparing for the MRCP(UK) at the Royal Postgraduate Medical School in London, the residents preparing for the Diplomate of Internal Medicine at Mount Sinai and the postgraduate students at the Kasturba Medical College preparing for the FRACP, MD (Int Med) and the Membership of the National Academy of Medical Sciences. Their advice and feedback have been invaluable in the evolution of the book and are gratefully acknowledged.

Readers who have any suggestions or constructive criticism to make which might help to improve subsequent editions of this book should write to Dr W. M. Chong, MRCP(UK), 8 Cissbury Ring South, Woodside Park, LONDON N12 7BE. All of these will be acknowledged, and subsequently credited where appropriate.

Questions

Case 1 ✓ ✓

A 55-year-old professor visited Singapore as an external university examiner and he progressively became confused and disorientated while roaming around the botanical gardens. He was found to be quite agitated. He was on antihistamines for hay fever. On examination he appeared drowsy and showed no signs of meningeal irritation, nor was the spleen palpable. His temperature was 38.5°C and the head CT scan was normal. He had atrial fibrillation, there was no neck rigidity, petechiae were noted over his body, the neurological examination did not localise any signs, and he was breathless. The blood investigations showed thrombocytopenia, hypoglycaemia, hyperkalaemia and metabolic acidosis. The ECG was normal with some premature ventricular ectopics. The CK and CKMB were normal.

Questions

Q1.1 **What is the diagnosis?**

Q1.2 **How would you treat this patient if he had presented with the same symptoms in England?**

Q1.3 **How would you approach this patient if his CK is above 1000 IU/l, his urine is black and the dipstick is positive?**

Q1.4 **He was discharged from hospital on erythromycin, for presumed chest infection, and terfenadine. The ECG showed a QRS duration of 0.4s on discharge. He died on the tarmac of the airport. What had happened?**

Case 2 ✓

A 45-year-old Indian toddy seller (*toddy* is a form of Indian alcohol) gave a three-month history of loose stools and weight loss of 3 kg. He had had several episodes of fainting.

Investigations showed:

Hb	13 g/dl
WCC	10×10^9/l
Serum bilirubin	19 µmol/l
Albumin	38 g/l
Alkaline phosphatase	132 IU/l
Aspartate transaminase	70 IU/l
Three-day faecal fat excretion	75 mmol/day
25 g oral D-xylose:	Recovery after 5 h

Questions

Q2.1   What is the likely diagnosis?
Q2.2   What are the possible underlying causes of this condition?
Q2.3   Suggest some useful investigations

Case 3

A 60-year-old *cordon bleu* chef who sustained an inferior infarct four years ago, had to stop at Stage 2 of the Bruce protocol because of precordial discomfort. The 12-lead ECG showed pathological (more then 2 mm) ST leads corresponding to the depression in the anterior descending artery.

Questions

Q3.1   What is the significance of the stress test?
Q3.2   When should one perform a coronary angiogram?
Q3.3   What is the difference between the sensitivity and specificity of a test?
Q3.4   What is the difference between a type I and a type II error?
Q3.5   What is syndrome X pertaining to insulin resistance?

Case 4

A 33-year-old Mir space flight controller staggered into casualty with pyrexia, ataxia, slurring of speech and drowsiness. There was no history of head injury or alcoholism, and the routine urine drug screen was negative. A CT scan was normal but the CSF showed:

Pressure	210 mm H_2O
Cells	83/mm^3 (80% polymorphs)
Protein	0.75 g/l
Glucose	2.1 mmol/l (blood glucose 4.3 mmol/l)

Questions

Q4.1   What is the diagnosis?
Q4.2   What investigations would you pursue?
Q4.3   What is the therapy?

Case 5

A child who was suspected of being abused was brought into casualty looking miserable and crying. Several blue marks were seen on his buttocks. Multiple fractures were noted on the X-ray films. On admission, his biochemical results showed a calcium serum level of 1.8 mmol/l, and an inorganic phosphate level of 0.8 mmol/l. The 25 hydroxyvitamin D$_3$ (25 OHD$_3$) was 26% of the reference sera.

Question

Q5.1   What are the possible diagnoses?

Case 6

A 37-year-old Algerian bus conductor had anterior pituitary failure secondary to an expanding acromegalic tumour. This was successfully treated by yttrium implants at the Hammersmith Hospital. He was started on cortisol and thyroxine. He felt better, but soon developed nocturia. At 9 a.m. the urinary osmolality was recorded as 333 mosmol/kg and the plasma osmolality was 294 mosmol/kg. He was not allowed water for eight hours, when the measurements were repeated. He had lost 4 kg in wight and the urine osmolarity was 239 mosmol/kg. The plasma osmolality was 300 mosmol/kg.

Question

Q6.1   What is the significance of these results and why did he develop nocturia?

Case 7

A 14-year-old Scottish boy with dysmorphic facies was treated with oral iron and injectable iron with no respite. The blood film was dimorphic, Hb 5 g/dl, MCHC 26 g/dl and MCV 65 fl.

Questions

Q7.1   What are the possible diagnoses and how would you investigate?
Q7.2   What is the management of this disorder?

Case 8 ✓

A 18-year-old student brought in an infant aged three weeks into the clinic after her partner told her that he had syphilis. The girl tested positive for syphilis but the child's results were:

    WR   Positive
    FTA   Positive
    FTA IgM   Positive

Question

Q8.1 Has the child got syphilis?

Case 9

A 19-year-old diabetic man had a plasma creatinine of 140 µmol/l. The urine production over 24 hours was 1200 ml, which contained 24 mmol of creatinine and 21 g of protein.

Questions

Q9.1 What has happened to the creatinine clearance?
Q9.2 This man presents 20 years later because of 'fatigue' and has not been complying well with the treatment prescribed. He is confused and has noticed occasional 'twitching' of his pectoral muscles. His mini mental test score is 5. The biochemical results suggest that he has uraemic encephalopathy. How will you manage him?
Q9.3 What is the relationship between low magnesium and hypocalcaemia?
Q9.4 What is aluminium toxicity?

Case 10 ✓

A 24-year-old Stanford MBA student complained of night sweats. Physical examination revealed some violaceous plaques on his chest but CXR showed bilateral hilar lymph node enlargement.

    Hb   13 g/dl
    WCC   9 × 10⁹/l
    ESR   56 mm in the first hour

Questions

Q10.1 What is the most likely diagnosis?
Q10.2 How would you establish the diagnosis?

Case 11

A 28-year-old Russian computer engineer with a past history of sun-burns and a rash over the face, visual blurring and arthralgia was referred by an obstetrician. She had been noted to behave bizarrely during social events and there was loss of fine movement over the right side of the body causing fumbling while playing the piano. Five years ago she had a DVT while on the oral contraceptive pill and has had four miscarriages at 15–17 weeks. An IUD was implanted a fortnight ago, after which she developed femoral vein thrombosis while on a heparin infusion:

Hb	10 g/dl
WCC	8×10^9/l (no abnormal cells noted)
Platelets	39×10^9
Creatinine clearance	120 ml/min
ANA	1 in 50
ENA	Negative
VDRL	Positive 1 in 1
Plasma sodium	145 mmol/l
Plasma potassium	4.6 mmol/l
Plasma urea	5 mmol/l

Questions

Q11.1 What is the diagnosis?
Q11.2 How would you advise the obstetrician in future pregnancies?
Q11.3 What is the neurological basis of her symptoms?

Case 12

A young lieutenant and five soldiers arrived at a base hospital appearing exhausted. A canister had exploded 300 yards from them, releasing a cloud of gas close to their vehicle during their foray into enemy territory. They all complained of abdominal pain.

One soldier collapsed and died from respiratory arrest. It transpired that none of them had had time to change into protective anti-personnel suits. On examination, all had increased respiratory secretion and pupillary constriction.

Questions

Q12.1 What happened and and how should it be handled?
Q12.2 What other insecticide is rapidly toxic?

Case 13

A 40-year-old insurance broker, who denied alcohol abuse, was hospitalised following a fall. She was described as ataxic and confused. On examination she was hyporeflexic, and nystagmus was present. The following investigations are obtained:

Head CT scan	Normal
CSF	Normal
Blood:	
Hb	12 g/dl
MCV	110 fl
WCC	$12 \times 10^9/l$
ESR	40 mm in the first hour

Questions

Q13.1 What is the diagnosis?
Q13.2 What investigations would you perform?
Q13.3 How should this be treated?

Case 14

A Russian computer hacker was noted to be blue and had clubbing of the hands. He underwent cardiac catheterisation:

	Pressure (mmHg)	O_2 saturation (%)
SVC	–	65
IVC	–	66
RA	5	66
RV	120/4	67
PA	145/146	67
Pulmonary capillary wedge	7	–
LV	120/0	78
FA	120/70	79

Questions

Q14.1 *What is the diagnosis?*

Q14.2 *What would your thoughts be if the catheterisation results were not present and a teenager presented with the same clinical picture and bilateral crackles?*

Q14.3 *What are the normal values for cardiac catheterisation data?*

Case 15

A 25-year-old nursing student was admitted to casualty at 2 a.m. with a headache after working in the Special Care Baby Unit the previous morning. She had woken up delirious and had collapsed in a semi-comatose state. She was febrile at 38°C, with marked neck rigidity, photophobia and a positive Kernig's sign. She had just returned from an holiday in Cameroon.

Questions

Q15.1 *What would be your immediate action?*

Q15.2 *What are the causes of hypoglycaemia?*

Q15.3 *How do you differentiate factitious from true hypoglycaemia?*

Case 16

A 4-year-old kindergarten child was diagnosed with a low IQ and, on examination, was found to have multiple teeth marks on his arms. He irritated his teacher by winking at her every five minutes, and threw his colour pencils around the room. He was noted to have spasticity and arthropathy. A subsequent bone marrow biopsy showed leukaemia. Plasma investigations showed:

Urea	4 mmol/l
Urate	0.8 mmol/l
Calcium	2.4 mmol/l
Phosphate	0.7 mmol/l

Questions

Q16.1 *What is the diagnosis?*

Q16.2 *If the patient is on mercaptopurine for leukaemia and one wanted to prevent a massive urate rise with a xanthine oxidase inhibitor, how would you titrate the dose of mercaptopurine?*

Case 17

A 32-year-old legal secretary complained of oligomenorrhoea and obesity. She had begun to shave with her boyfriend's razor. He had noticed that she had grown hairs on her chest and became more aggressive. Investigations showed:

9 a.m. cortisol	480 nmol/l
Testosterone	6 nmol/l (normal range 0.8–3.1)
LH	7.1 IU/l
FSH	2.8 IU/l
Prolactin	381 mU (normal range < 360)
SHBG	23 nmol/l (normal range 46–110)

After 0.5 mg dexamethasone six hourly for 48 hours:

9 a.m. cortisol	< 70 nmol/l
Testosterone	5 nmol/l

Question

Q17.1 What further investigations are indicated and what is the diagnosis?

Case 18

A 34-year-old formula one driver underwent an emergency laparotomy after a crash in Monte Carlo three years ago. His blood count revealed a platelet count of $503 \times 10^9/l$.

Questions

Q18.1 Why is the platelet count deranged?

Q18.2 What are the other causes of such a high elevation of platelets?

Case 19

A 23-year-old Filipina cocktail waitress was admitted as an emergency for pain over the right hypochondrium. The pain was worse on inspiration, Murphy's sign was negative and she began to retch. Seven weeks ago, she had had a casual affair (she was on oral contraception) and subsequently developed pustules all over her body, which cleared. Her male friend had a clear urethral discharge and arthritis of the right knee.

On examination she was febrile at 37.4°C, breathless and tender over the right hypochondrium. A rub was audible over the liver, no visceromegaly was detectable and she had a greyish white vaginal discharge. Her vital signs were normal and the symptoms subsided over the next few days while she was taking a course of antibiotics.

Questions

Q19.1 What is the diagnosis?
Q19.2 How would you treat this patient?

Case 20

A 45-year-old Bosnian woman with chronic glomerulonephritis developed headache after 12 years of haemodialysis. She was diagnosed as HIV positive seven years ago. Her past medical history is significant for PCP and a total CD4 count of 90. She is currently on pyrimethamine and sulphadiazine. She has been febrile at 38°C and the 'light hurt her eyes'. There are no focal neurological deficits. LP, after a normal CT, reveals five white cells. The cryptococcal antigen is positive 1:153 and the India ink test is positive. Investigations showed microscopic haematuria and a Hb of 19 g/dl.

Questions

Q20.1 What is your diagnosis?
Q20.2 What is the importance of diagnosing the cysts early?
Q20.3 What further investigations should be performed?

Case 21

A 45-year-old 'bug' (remote sensor) designer, who does not smoke, developed a nocturnal cough. The cough is exacerbated by cold. Investigation revealed:

    FEV$_1$ 2.3 litre (predicted 3–4)
    FVC   3.8 litre (predicted 5–6)
    FEV$_1$/FVC 61%

The methacoline provocation test revealed that the concentration producing a 21% drop in FEV$_1$ = 1 mg/ml (normal > 4 mg/ml).

Questions

Q21.1   What diagnosis is indicated by the test of lung function?
Q21.2   What may have caused this disorder?

Case 22

A 55-year-old Belgian woman was examined for aching of the neck and
back for a year. She has had early morning stiffness for an hour each day
for the last six months. Four months prior to her appointment she
noticed bruising over all her extremities. Haematological investigations
revealed:

Hb	10 g/dl
WCC	4×10^9/l
Platelets	300×10^9/l
ESR	135 mm in the first hour
Sodium	138 nmol/l
Potassium	4.9 nmol/
Urea	16 mmol/l
Creatinine	300 mmol/l
Phosphate	2.3 mmol/l
Alkaline phosphatase	70 IU/l
Bilirubin	7 μmol/l

Protein electrophoresis shows a drop in all the immunoglobulins, X-ray
examination of the spine demonstrates osteoporosis and the bone scan is
normal.

Questions

Q22.1   What is the diagnosis?
Q22.2   How would you treat this disorder?

Case 23

A 30-year-old abbot of a monastery had just given a darshan (spiritual
teaching) to his followers. He walked through the paddy fields and was
fed rice and vegetables by a wood cutter. He developed abdominal
discomfort and became unable to walk, having to lie down. He also
described blurring of vision and his speech was slurred. Examination
revealed diplopia, ataxia and photophobia. He did not give a history of
taking any drugs which may have precipitated an acute dystonic reaction, nor was there a flesh wound to suggest tetanus.

Questions

Q23.1 What is the diagnosis?
Q23.2 Does a past history of recovery from tetanus confer lifelong immunity?
Q23.3 Is there another toxin one should consider in the region?

Case 24

A 50-year-old illegal immigrant from Hong Kong who was working in a Chinese restaurant in Soho, became temporarily blind while in police custody. On examination, he had an abdominal mass and pedal oedema.

Hb	20 g/dl
PCV	0.6%
MCV	103 fl
Platelets	50×10^9/l
Albumin	15 g/l

Question

Q24.1 What is the diagnosis?

Case 25

A 45-year-old Bosnian window cleaner underwent cardiac catheter-isation for breathlessness. Pressures (mmHg) were:

RA	5
RV	78/4
PA	78/30
Wedge	mean of 18
LV	110/2

Questions

Q25.1 What is wrong with her and what is the treatment?
Q25.2 When does one cardiovert electrically for atrial fibrillation?
Q25.3 What if the patient in atrial fibrillation complains of severe abdominal pain with no guarding?
Q25.4 How do you calculate pulmonary vascular resistance?

Case 26

A 35-year-old Hindu priest of the Sankara sect complained of breathlessness for the past week. He noticed that his dyspnoea increased as he walked deeper into the Ganges for his morning purification ceremony and he had difficulty clambering on to the river bank. On examination, he appeared fit. His pulse was 80/min and regular. There were no signs of the use of accessory muscles, but there was bilateral winging of the scapulae with no sensory loss. A tensilon test was performed, with full cardiorespiratory resuscitative equipment available. It was found to be normal and there was no history of the weakness improving on increased activity, ruling out the Eaton–Lambert syndrome.

Question

Q26.1 Why is he breathless?

Case 27

A 60-year-old United Nations consultant working in Bhutan suffered a cardiac arrest but was successfully resuscitated. Five days later, the following results were obtained:

Serum bilirubin	85 µmol/l
Serum alkaline phosphatase	250 IU/l
Serum aspartate aminotransferase	2600 IU/l

Question

Q27.1 What is the likely diagnosis?

Case 28

A 55-year-old physiotherapist complained of proximal weakness while demonstrating to patients who had back problems how to carry weights safely. This was a prolapsed disc rehabilitation class. Her results are:

Hb	13 g/dl
MCH	30 g/dl
MCV	86 fl
Sodium	128 mmol/l
Potassium	4 mmol/l
Cholesterol	10 mmol/l

Questions

Q28.1 *What is the diagnosis and why is the sodium so low?*
Q28.2 *How would you screen for this disorder?*
Q28.3 *What is 'apathetic thyrotoxicosis'?*

Case 29

A 15-year-old premenarchal South African girl previously diagnosed with β-thalassaemia major was admitted for sudden breathlessness. Although she appeared grey compared with her peers, the pulmonary function tests were normal:

Hb   7.8 g/dl
Fe   33 µmol/l
TIBC 82 µmol/l

Questions

Q29.1 *What are the possible causes of her heart failure?*
Q29.2 *What is the haematological diagnostic profile of thalassaemia minor?*

Case 30

A 49-year-old professor of chemical engineering, who has a large collection of stray cats, complained of feeling sick for the past week. On examination, the cervical lymph nodes were hot. He had a row with his current girlfriend who is a literature lecturer at another university when she found out that he was going out with his PhD student. A provisional diagnosis of infectious mononucleosis was made: Hb 14 g/dl, WCC 9×10^9/l (24% lymphocytes with no atypical cells). A heterophile antibody test was done:

No absorption on ox red cells: Agglutination with sheep RBC
After absorption on ox red cells: Agglutination with sheep RBC
After absorption on guinea pig kidney: No agglutination with sheep RBC

Questions

Q30.1 *What do you deduce from these results?*
Q30.1 *What is a possible diagnosis?*

Case 31

A 76-year-old Swiss police officer has visual blurring, which is being treated at the main hospital:

Sodium	138 mmol/l
Potassium	3.2 mmol/l
Bicarbonate	4 mmol/l
Chloride	125 mmol/l
$PaCO_2$	2 kPa
pH	7.0

Questions

Q31.1 For what is he being treated?
Q31.2 What are the other causes of this biochemical profile?

Case 32

A 40-year-old barrister with rheumatoid arthritis found it difficult to represent her client in a case of theft, because of breathlessness. On examination, she had finger clubbing and basal crackles. The chest radiogram demonstrated basal shadowing and the results of pulmonary function tests were:

FEV_1	1.79 litre (predicted 2–3)
FVC	2.2 litre (predicted 2.5–3.5)
FEV_1/FVC	81%
TLC	3.6 litre (predicted 4–6)
Transfer coefficient for carbon monoxide (TLCO)	1 mmol min^{-1} kPa^{-1} l^{-1} (predicted 1.3–2)

Questions

Q32.1 What is the cause of her breathlessness?
Q32.2 How would you confirm this diagnosis?
Q32.3 What are the causes of reduced gas transfer (TLCO)?
Q32.4 What are the causes of increased gas transfer?

Case 33

A 47-year-old gifted violinist who had attended the rheumatology clinic since the age of 26 when he was a student at the Royal Academy, was diagnosed with SLE. He had been on steroids much of the time. He has managed to reduce his steroid dose to 5 mg daily. However he sustained a spontaneous vertebral crush fracture while on a tour to New York and cracked five ribs during a fall after a recital.

An echocardiogram suggested right heart failure. The ECG demonstrated right ventricular strain. A recent lung function test before the fall showed a VC of 2, an FEV_1 of 1.6, a low transfer factor and a residual volume of one litre. The CXR confirmed the fractures, but there was no pneumothorax and no plate atelectasis. Routine urinary tests revealed proteinuria and RBCs.

Questions

Q33.1 How would you manage him assuming that he needs an operation?

Q33.2 What is the significance of the lung function test?

Case 34

A 44-year-old Chinese takeaway owner was found wielding a knife at one of his customer who arrested him as he was an off duty detective. The family pleaded with the officer not to take him away as he is currently on chlorpromazine and has just been released from the local psychiatric hospital. His temperature was 36°C. He was, however, hospitalised and the following results were obtained:

T_4	200 nmol/l
THUT	160
FTI	198 nmol/l
T_3	5 nmol/l
TSH	3 mU/l

Questions

Q34.1 What is the diagnosis?

Q34.2 What other conditions may produce this biochemical profile?

Case 35

A consultant psychiatrist, who underwent a successful hip operation for a motor vehicle accident in Los Angeles, was making a splendid recovery until the fourth postoperative night. She shouted and complained that the wall was moving towards her and that there was an assassin hiding under her bed. Auscultation did not reveal any signs and there were no petechiae seen on her eyelids. The blood results were normal apart from an MCV of 110 fl, but she showed no signs suggestive of impending shock.

A CT scan of the head was normal.

Questions

Q35.1 *What is the diagnosis?*
Q35.2 *What is the treatment?*
Q35.3 *What questions would you ask her?*

Case 36

A 36-year-old Ethiopian maxillo-facial surgeon was admitted following collapse and a fit following a hot afternoon ward round. She has a history of five blackouts over the past 20 years, three of which were followed by fits. Each episode had been preceded by exercise or a meal. On examination, she is neurologically normal. The pulse is 60 beats/min and regular with a slow upstroke. Peripheral pulses are normal. On auscultation, she has a loud ejection systolic murmur all over the precordium, which radiates to the carotids. The ECG shows sinus rhythm and left ventricular hypertrophy. Echocardiography demonstrates a normal aortic valve.

Questions

Q36.1 *What is the diagnosis?*
Q36.2 *What would you consider if she presented with rectal bleeding and aortic stenosis?*
Q36.3 *What if this patient has supravalvular aortic stenosis, a highly developed sense of musical ability, hypercalcaemia and a relatively borderline IQ?*

Case 37

A 23-year-old Danish student of economics presented with a history of leg weakness and backache. He has a birthmark on his right axilla and is on anti-hypertension medication. After the CT scan of the head (which was normal), an l.p. showed the following CSF findings:

        Cells   3 lymphocytes/mm^3
        Protein   4.5 g/l
        Glucose   3.9 mmol/l (blood glucose 4.7 mmol/l)

Questions

Q37.1 What did the myelogram show?
Q37.2 What other pathology may be associated with this condition?
Q37.3 What is the cause of his visual difficulties?

Case 38

A 22-year-old girl was admitted following a row with her boyfriend, when she threw his belongings out of a fifth floor flat window. She appeared febrile and arterial blood gas revealed:

PaO_2 14 kPa
$PaCO_2$ 3.6 kPa
pH   7.49

Question

Q38.1 What has happened and what is the treatment?

Case 39

A 34-year-old asthmatic Sikh physician regularly takes valium for insomnia. She is being seen by a psychologist for 'melancholia' because of unrequited love. She noted blurring of her vision while reading an ECG during a ward round. She was admitted for malaise and headache. Her BP was 182/126 mmHg and there was no papilloedema. She was successfully treated with nifedipine, frusemide and oral diazoxide.

A subsequent IVP was normal and the peripheral renin level was $3481 \, pg \, ml^{-1} h^{-1}$, urea 12 mmol/l, GFR 50 ml/min and urine microscopy showed no abnormality. There was a proteinuria of 1.5 g/day. Two weeks later, her renin level had doubled and the GFR had dropped to 32 ml/min. Several months later, she returned complaining of fine silky hair growing over her face.

Questions

Q39.1 What was the original diagnosis and what changes occurred after therapy?
Q39.2 What is the significance of the hair growth?

Case 40

A Polish nurse was treated for macrocytic anaemia with vitamin B_{12} when the Hb was 7.5 g/dl. There was a 10% reticulocytosis on day 5, but despite the twice weekly i.m. vitamin B_{12}, the Hb failed to rise above 10 g/dl.

Questions

Q40.1   What was the reason for the failure of the Hb to rise?
Q40.2   What are the other causes of macrocytosis?

Case 41

A 77-year-old French gentleman used to be an army officer in Burma. He has returned to Yangon as a diplomatic attaché intermittently for several years. He presented to his GP with generalised itching. This was treated and it improved. He then underwent extensive investigations for unexplained weight loss and abdominal pain. Gastroscopy revealed no abnormality. He was admitted several times for feeling generally sick and complained of a constant pain in the stomach. He is reassured repeatedly that this is not cancer. The serum amylase is normal and he gives a four-month history of intermittent non-bloody diarrhoea. He has episodes of an itchy eruption on the back. There are no haematological indices suggestive of polycythaemia but the eosinophil count is high. He has lost 13 kg in weight and the abdomen is generally tender. He was afebrile.

Questions

Q41.1   What is the diagnosis?
Q41.2   What investigations would you perform?
Q41.3   How is this treated?

Case 42

A 22-year-old Spanish secretary with recurrent loin pain passes some urinary granules. These granules were analysed in the laboratory. They were found to comprise predominantly ammonium hydrogen urate stones. Her pregnancy test is positive.

Q42.1 What are the likely causes of these stones and their therapy?
Q42.2 What drugs are relatively safe in pregnancy?

Case 43

A 45-year-old commercial pilot, who had just flown back from Poona, believed that he had contracted the plague as it was supposedly endemic in that area. He presented with a two-week history of malaise, diarrhoea and myalgia. He also complained of numbness and loss of manual dexterity of the right arm, which interfered with his control of the aircraft. He had a cough producing yellow sputum and a blotchy red rash over his chest. CXR demonstrated bilateral patchy pneumonitis in both lower zones. He had no dermatological signs. He was started on tetracycline for presumed plague. He was also on metronidazole for amoebiasis, but broke quarantine and left the hospital. He recovered over the next three weeks. Investigation showed:

Hb	8 g/dl
Reticulocyte count	5%
MCV	110 fl
WCC	9×10^9/l

Questions

Q43.1 What is the diagnosis and how would you confirm it?
Q43.2 What is the treatment?
Q43.3 He celebrated the news that he does not have the plague by drinking some vodka. He began to sweat, retch and collapsed. What had occurred?

Case 44

A 34-year-old cat burglar who fell off his motorbike, injured his neck. It later came to light that he had a past history of severe back pain associated with poor cervical mobility. MRI revealed that he had fractured his neck but the cord was miraculously undamaged. He was treated with steroids to reduce cord oedema. The crash helmet was not removed in casualty as it supported his neck, and the neurosurgeons stabilised his neck by an open procedure. He had breathlessness and a pneumothorax was ruled out.

The results of the lung function tests were: FEV$_1$ 2.9 litres and FVC 3 litres.

Questions

Q44.1 *What underlying problem does this man have?*
Q44.2 *What bedside tests may be performed to follow up the progression of this disorder?*
Q44.3 *How do you analyse back pain?*
Q44.4 *What is DISH?*
Q44.5 *How would you manage this disorder?*

Case 45

A 35-year-old man who was on medication for obsessive compulsive behaviour was admitted following a convulsion. He regularly attends parties and takes ecstasy tablets but reassures everyone that he is well prepared for its side effects. The EEG was normal, the serum sodium was 110 mmol/l, plasma osmolality 240 mosmol/kg, and the urinary specific gravity was 1.000.

Questions

Q45.1 *What is the likely diagnosis?*

Case 46

A 55-year-old Croatian aeroplane repair maintenance engineer presented with severe Raynaud's phenomenon and breathlessness. He also noticed progressive dysphagia and fever. The following blood results were obtained:

Albumin	36 g/l
Globulin	41 g/l
IgA	3 g/l
IgG	11 g/l
IgM	8.5 g/l
Alkaline phosphatase	1350 IU/l
SGPT	36 IU/l
Bilirubin	22 µmol/l

Question

Q46.1 What is the diagnosis and may his occupation have any relevance?

Case 47

A 45-year-old Israeli security officer underwent cardiac catheterisation following several episodes of nocturnal breathlessness. The pressures (mmHg) were:

Mean RA	4
RV	25/6
Pulmonary artery	26/6
Mean pulmonary wedge	14
V	200/14
Aorta	120/80

Questions

Q47.1 What are the possible diagnoses?
Q47.2 What is the relationship of the outflow gradient to the prognosis?

Case 48

A 25-year-old priest collapsed in the pulpit while conducting mass. He was incoherent, complained of a headache and photophobia and had mild disk swelling on fundoscopy. He underwent splenectomy several years ago for hereditary spherocytosis. On examination, he had a well healed abdominal scar and some leg ulcers. CT scan of the head was normal:

CSF:		
	Pressure	290 mm H_2O
	Protein	2 g/l
	Cells	200 cells/mm^3 (90%) polymorphs
	Glucose	1.5 mmol/l
	Gram stain	Gram-positive diplococci
Blood:		
	Hb	10 g/dl
	WCC	18 × 10^9/l, 13% lymphocytes
	ESR	84 mm in the first hour
	Glucose	6 mmol/l

Questions

Q48.1 What is the diagnosis and what therapy should be instituted?
Q48.2 What is his prognosis?

Case 49

A 36-year-old merchant banker presented with backache and pelvic pain. On investigation, X-ray examinationof the spine showed osteoporotic changes and medullary calcification of the kidney. Investigations showed:

Urine pH	7–6.4
Three-day faecal fat excretion	14 g/day
D-xylose absorption	1 g excreted in 5 h after 5 g orally
Blood urea	6 mmol/l
Serum calcium	2 mmol/l
Serum phosphate	1.4 mmol/l
Serum albumin	45 g/l
Arterial pH	7.4

Questions

Q49.1 What are the diagnoses?
Q49.2 How would you confirm your suspicion?
Q49.3 What is Bartter's syndrome?

Case 50

A 36-year-old Latin teacher was receiving therapy for cancer of the prostate. The diagnosis was made following a routinely elevated PSA and confirmed by a tissue biopsy. He developed gynaecomastia and swelling of the legs.

Question

Q50.1 What drug did he receive and what alternatives are there?

Case 51

A 20-year-old Down's patient who is anaemic presented with breathlessness. He is on long-term phenytoin for long-standing epilepsy. For a few years he has had episodes of backache and loss of appetite, when he became jaundiced (with dark urine). This recovered in 10 days with no therapy. Investigation shows:

Hb	4 g/dl
MCV	110 fl
WCC	$2 \times 10^9/l$
Blood film	Normal
Platelets	$50 \times 10^9/l$

Questions

Q51.1 What is the diagnosis?

Case 52

A 17-year-old student who had just returned from Goa was admitted for three days of non-bloody diarrhoea, fever, vomiting and headache. She has been sexually active and has a past history of gonorrhoea and completed treatment at the STD clinic a year ago. She was menstruating four days prior to admission. The entire group had taken prophylactic antimalarials for the prescribed period but none had similar symptoms. She was delirious, febrile at 38°C, flushed and had bilateral conjunctivitis. Her skin was diffusely erythematous with a 'macular-like sunburn'. Her BP was 78 mmHg systolic; the diastolic pressure was unrecordable. The pulse rate was 140 per minute. The lungs were clear. Investigations showed:

Hb	14 g/dl
WCC	$18 \times 10^9/l$ (80% neutrophils)
Platelets	$50 \times 10^9/l$
Plasma sodium	130 mmol/l
Plasma potassium	3 mmol/l
Plasma urea	17 mmol/l
Plasma creatinine	230 µmol/l
Blood glucose	7 mmol/l

LP (lumbar puncture) shows clear fluid containing four red cells, one lymphocyte and a CSF glucose of 5 mmol/l. Cultures of blood and stool were repeatedly negative. A high vaginal swab grew *Staphylococcus aureus*.

Questions

Q52.1 What is the diagnosis?

Q52.2   What is the management?
Q52.3   What are the criteria for diagnosing this condition?

Case 53

A 35-year-old truck driver had proteinuria of 1.2 g/day. He noted 'ants gathering' where he passed urine whilein the Australian outback. The other blood results were plasma pH 7.35, uric acid clearance of 16 ml/min (normal 6–8 ml/min) and a plasma phosphate of 0.6 mmol/l. The maximum urine acidity after a 0.1 g/kg body weight load of ammonium chloride was 5.5. The maximum urinary concentration after dehydration and pitressin was 499 mmol/l. Chromatography of the urine showed aminoaciduria; electrophoresis showed a little albumin and increased quantities of β_2-microglobulin.

Question

Q53.1   What is the diagnosis?

Case 54

A 76-year-old Welsh woman schoolteacher who smokes 40 cigarettes presented with a four-month history of haemoptysis. She had finger clubbing and the CXR demonstrated a cavitating lesion in the left lower lobe, with some right upper lobe opacity and an elevated right hemidiaphragm. She had been injected with steroids by her son who was currently a medical student in Germany. He had read that this would help stress and malaise. Investigation showed:

    Calcium   3.8 mmol/l
    Phosphate   1.2 mmol/l

Questions

Q54.1   What is the probable diagnosis?
Q54.2   How does one treat hypercalcaemia?
Q54.3   What are the other causes of hypercalcaemia?

Case 55

A 35-year-old architect was admitted for control of BP of 240/140 mmHg and retinopathy. He was given oral nifedipine 20 mg eight-hourly and was initially told to bite a 10 mg nifedipine capsule and to swallow it. The BP was monitored carefully to prevent any sudden drop, since this may cause cerebral insufficiency and cause a stroke in the watershed zone. He was then started on sodium nitroprusside (after a history of asthma was obtained), as this was not effective in BP control.

His BP was stabilised and normalised with a combination of calcium channel blockers and bendrofluazide. However, he developed fresh haemorrhages in the ensuing week after discharge, but he reported excellent BP control which was confirmed by his 24-hour BP monitor. For unexplained reasons his results went missing.

Questions

Q55.1 *Suggest other diagnoses*
Q55.2 *What are the causes of secondary hypertension?*
Q55.3 *How would you diagnose renal artery stenosis, apart from attempting to listen to a bruit?*
Q55.4 *What are the dangers of sodium nitroprusside use?*

Case 56

A 22-year-old financial executive presented to his general practitioner with abdominal pain, tenderness over the hypochondrium, poorly healing scars on the leg, fever and canary-yellow sclera. There was bile in the urine, and liver function tests showed:

Plasma bilirubin	130 μmol/l
Serum alkaline phosphatase	208 IU/l
Plasma alanine aminotransferase (SGPT)	40 IU/l
Hb	10 g/dl
MCHC	39 g/dl
MCV	88 fl (seen in the blood film with the morphology smaller and darker than normal)

Coombs' test was negative, and the reticulocyte count 10%.

Questions

Q56.1 *What is the diagnosis?*
Q56.2 *What additional history is needed?*

Case 57

An 18-year-old student of herbal medicine who is being treated for Crohn's disease has the following blood count:

Hb   9.3 g/dl
Reticulocytes   5%

The blood film shows fragmentation and Heinz bodies in abundance after incubation for 48 hours.

Question

Q57.1 What is the reason for the deranged blood film?

Case 58

In a 38-year-old Swedish watchmaker, a former alcoholic but now an active participant of Alcoholics Anonymous, cardiac catheterisation reveals normal coronary arteries, and mild mitral and tricuspid regurgitation. The following are the angiographic measurements of his left ventricular function:

End systolic volume   155 ml
End diastolic volume   183 ml
Ejection fraction   16% (with no regional wall motion abnormality)

Question

Q58.1 What is the diagnosis and what should be done?

Case 59

A 22-year-old dental student at King's College was seen in the clinic with a six-week history of fatigue and migratory pain in the joints and muscles. Her smile had appeared crooked to her classmates that morning. She jogs regularly in Richmond Park and is a keen photographer. There was no past history of note except an annular rash over her right breast which disappeared spontaneously. There was also pain and swelling over the right knee. Investigations revealed:

Hb	12 g/dl
Urate level	0.6 mmol/l
WCC	$7 \times 10^9/l$
ESR	50 mm in the first hour
Rheumatoid factor	Negative
ANA	Negative

Questions

Q59.1 What is she suffering from and how is this confirmed?
Q59.2 What would the CSF show?
Q59.3 How is this treated?
Q59.4 What is the Lofgren syndrome?

Case 60

A 46-year-old poacher, who is a keen deer hunter, was investigated because of abdominal pain, which ultrasonography revealed to be due to kidney stones. Investigations reveal:

Serum calcium	2.9 mmol/l
Serum albumin	39 g/l
Serum phosphate	1.3 mmol/l
Urinary calcium excretion	9 mmol/24 hours

Following oral hydrocortisone therapy every eight hours for 10 days, the fasting calcium was 2.5 mmol/l

Questions

Q60.1 What is the explanation for the biochemical changes?
Q60.2 What are the situations requiring corticosteroid treatment in sarcoidosis?
Q60.3 How would you diagnose sarcoidosis?

Case 61

A 30-year-old basket ball player underwent cosmetic surgery for gynaecomastia three years ago. He is 2 m tall (pubis to heel distance 97 cm and pubis to head 94 cm) and has an arm span of 1.95 m. He and his wife are being investigated for infertility. Investigations revealed:

Serum testosterone   5 nmol/l (normal range 10–30)
LH   30 U/l (normal range < 6)
FSH   43 U/l (normal range < 6)
Buccal smear   Positive for Barr bodies

Questions

Q61.1   What is the diagnosis and the treatment?
Q61.2   What is the incidence of this disorder?

Case 62

A 45-year-old accountant complained of severe itching all over his body. Investigations revealed:

Hb   20 g/dl
PCV   60%
MCV   78 fl
WCC $12 \times 10^9/l$

The differential count was normal. The blood film showed a few nucleated cells. The biochemical parameters were normal.

Questions

Q62.1   What is the diagnosis?
Q62.2   How would you confirm the diagnosis?
Q62.3   What are the therapeutic options?

Case 63

A 22-year-old Kurdish lawyer noticed clumsiness as he handled papers in court and sudden blurring of the right eye. He had had some dragging of the left foot a year ago, which resolved. His family urged him to make the pilgrimage to Bernadette's grotto at Lourdes. He refused, explaining that they may all be guilty of the *'post hoc ergo propter hoc* fallacy'. There was a central zone of blurring which did not improve with a change of glasses. Visual-evoked responses show:

Left   P100   95 ms (amplitude 13 mV with the upper limit of normal 108 ms)
Right   P100   130 ms (amplitude 5 μV)

Question

Q63.1 What is the cause of the visual problem?

Case 64

A 26-year-old tourist returning from India with chronic renal failure, who had been prescribed a vegetarian diet by an Aryuvedic practitioner (herbalist), presented in an emaciated state. The blood urea was 14 mmol/l and the serum creatinine 400 µmol/l.

Questions

Q64.1 What is the reason for the biochemical picture seen?
Q64.2 In what other conditions may this disparity be found?

Case 65

A 17-year-old stable boy with asthma, fever and cough with worsening sputum production has a CXR showing bilateral upper zone shadowing, which was not present in the last series taken 4 years previously. Investigations showed:

Hb   14 g/dl
WCC $9 \times 10^9/l$ (60% neutrophils, 13% eosinophils, 19% lymphocytes and 8% monocytes)
ESR   66 mm in the first hour

Sputum was negative for AAFB (acid alcohol fast bacilli) on four occasions.

Questions

Q65.1 What are the possible causes of the CXR changes?
Q65.2 What are the features of an acute severe attack of asthma?
Q65.3 How would you manage an acute attack of asthma?

Case 66

A 30-year-old travel writer presented with pain in both ankles after a trip to Equador. He also complained of urinary frequency with suprapubic discomfort occurring two weeks ago, while in Lima. He also had acute fever, diarrhoea and abdominal pain. The stools did not contain blood or mucus and these symptoms settled in three days. He attributed it to some tribal food he ate but he denied consuming goat's milk. He also denies extramarital intercourse. Examination revealed an ill man with a temperature of 37.9°C, with mild bilateral conjunctivitis, a left sided pleural rub and exquisitely tender ankle joints. There was also tenderness over the right iliac fossa but no palpable mass. Rectal examination was normal and sigmoidoscopy revealed some hyperaemia. Investigations revealed a normal blood film. Thick and thin films were performed three times to exclude malaria. The CXR was normal. Investigations showed:

Hb	12 g/dl
ESR	80 mm/first hour
WCC	14 × 10⁹/l (neutrophil leucocytosis)
Sodium	140 mmol/l
Potassium	3.3 mmol/l
Bicarbonate	30 mmol/l
Creatinine	100 μmol/l

Questions

Q66.1   What is the diagnosis?
Q66.2   What organisms are implicated?
Q66.3   Is this a sexually transmitted disease?
Q66.4   How do you analyse a joint aspirate?

Case 67

A 17-year-old South American student who was backpacking through France gave a history of palpitations and breathlessness, which had been worsening for the past six weeks. He had a headache and felt disorientated while visiting the Louvre. He collapsed and was admitted to hospital with symptoms of chest discomfort. Doppler echo demonstrated dilatation of all the chambers of the heart, with moderate tricuspid and mitral regurgitation. The ECG showed diffuse non-specific changes. Subsequent cardiac biopsy showed that this was compatible with viral cardiomyopathy. He is teetotal and denied the use of cocaine. The headache worsened and the CSF and blood tests showed:

CSF:
Pressure	180 mm H_2O
Proteins	0.38 g/l
Cells	34/mm³ lymphocytes
Glucose	5 mmol/l

Blood:
Hb   13 g/dl
WCC   4 × 10⁹/l (50% lymphocytes)
Glucose   5 mmol/l
CKMB   Normal

Questions

Q67.1 What is the diagnosis?
Q67.2 What other organisms may cause this picture?
Q67.3 What less common disorder may produce a similar picture?

Case 68

A 30-year-old physician's assistant who works in the operating theatre and had recently started on oral contraceptives, developed jaundice with pruritis. Several weeks after commencing the oral contraceptives, she was noted to have an icteric appearance. She gave no history of exposure to halothane, blood transfusion, or sharp injuries. She was taking no other medication, had adequate titres of protection from hepatitis B by vaccination and drank only social quantities of alcohol. On examination, no hepatomegaly was detectable and the CXR was unremarkable. The results were:

Hb	11 g/dl
MCV	80 fl
WCC	10 × 10⁹/l
Differential count	Normal
ESR	17 mm/h
Serum urea and electrolytes	normal
Serum alkaline phosphatase	85 IU/l
Total protein	67 g/l
Serum albumin	35 g/l
Serum calcium	2.4 mmol/l
SGOT	40 IU/l
Serum hydroxybutyrate dehydrogenase	113 IU/l
Urine analysis	Bile +++

Questions

Q68.1 What is the diagnosis?
Q68.2 How will you confirm it?
Q68.3 What is the prognosis?

Case 69

A telephonist at Sotheby's, who has had a systolic murmur all her life, underwent cardiac catheterisation. She had several documented episodes of palpitations, which disappeared when she stopped drinking Turkish coffee each morning. Investigations showed:

Right atrial pressure	7/0 mmHg
Right ventricular pressure	64/4 mmHg
Main pulmonary artery pressure	22/10 mmHg
Oxygen saturations:	
SVC	70%
Right atrium	86%
Right ventricle	83%
Pulmonary artery	81%

Questions

Q69.1 What is the diagnosis?
Q69.2 What would a CXR show?

Case 70

A 35-year-old Sicilian fisherman is seen in the rheumatology clinic because of a five-week history of arthritis intermittently affecting his legs. He has no tenderness of the sacroiliac joints but has complaints of intermittent diarrhoea and steatorrhoea (the stools resemble the colour of the old edition of the Bailey and Love textbook of surgery belonging to his brother who studies medicine). Small effusions were observed in both knees and a small bowel biopsy shows PAS positive material in the lamina propria of the intestines. He was found to be HLA B27 positive.

Questions

Q70.1 What is the diagnosis?
Q70.2 How should his arthritis be treated?
Q70.3 How do you classify diarrhoea?

Case 71

A 21-year-old legal secretary has been on chronic medication for convulsions. She was admitted for backache and was described as looking much older than her age. Investigations showed:

Blood urea	4 mmol/l
Serum albumin	43 g/l
Serum calcium	2 mmol/l
Serum inorganic phosphate	0.8 mmol/l
Plasma alkaline phosphatase	179 IU/l
Plasma	25-OHD$_3$ (33% of standard reference sera)

Questions

Q71.1 What is the diagnosis and how does this condition occur?

Case 72

A 35-year-old boxer walked into his manager's office one day carrying both antique rolling doors after smashing through them, apologising that he had not seen them. This seem to coincide with a sudden loss of skill. He used to be adept at dodging punches. He denied taking anabolic steroids and complained of paraesthesia and numbness over the hand. His GTT (after 75 g oral glucose) was:

Time (min)	Venous glucose (mmol/l)	GH (mU/l)
0	8	13
30	14	18
60	14.5	20
90	13.9	42
120	12.5	26

Questions

Q72.1 What are the diagnoses?
Q72.2 What happens to the GFR, the phosphate and the urinary calcium level?
Q72.3 What are the causes of death in this disorder?

Case 73

A 33-year-old lorry driver had several episodes of loss of control and paraesthesia over the left side of the body. He also noticed purpura on the body. Investigations showed:

BP	180/110 mmHg
Hb	8 g/dl
WCC	$11 \times 10^9/l$
Platelets	$50 \times 10^9/l$
Reticulocytes	4%
Plasma urea	40 mmol/l
Plasma sodium	125 mmol/l
Plasma potassium	6.3 mmol/l

The blood film showed microspherocytes ++ and red cell fragments ++.

Question

Q73.1   What possible diagnoses would you consider?

Case 74

A doctor working in an overcrowded prison was surprised when four out of five patients, who shared the same cell, developed flu-like symptoms, jaundice, nausea and vomiting. They had eaten the same meal as all of the other inmates of the island prison, and all denied sharing needles. There was no history of intimate contact, no history of illicit drugs or sharing a cache of 'special food', and records showed all of the five to be HBsAg negative.

One of the patients died suddenly following convulsions after complaining that the light hurt his eyes. The body was taken to the mainland coroner's laboratory for an autopsy. On examination there was no organomegaly and fundoscopy appeared normal, but petechiae were seen on the legs. The results of blood investigations showed:

Hb	13 g/dl
MCV	110 fl
WCC	$22 \times 10^9/l$ (80% neutrophils)
Platelets	$100 \times 10^9/l$
Bicarbonate	14 mmol/l
Glucose	7 mmol/l
PTTK	40 s (normal range 24–36)
PT (first test)	18 s (control 14 s)
PT (repeat test)	17 s (control 13 s)
Potassium	5 mmol/l
Urea	22 mmol/l
Bilirubin	90 µmol/l
SGOT	130 IU/l

Alkaline phosphatase	188 mmol/l
Albumin	38 g/l

Urinalysis results were:

Protein	+++++
RBC	+++
Bile	+++
Urobilinogen	++
CSF protein	0.6 g/l
Glucose	4.6 mmol/l (with lymphocytic pleocytosis)

Questions

Q74.1 What is the diagnosis?
Q74.2 How would you confirm it?
Q74.3 What is the prognosis?

Case 75

A 35-year-old female glassblower from Tipperary gave a four-month history of breathlessness and dry cough. She was well prior to this with no other pathology. Clubbing and dyspnoea with central cyanosis were noted. On auscultation, fine crackles were noted over the lung bases with a palpable P_2. She had surgery for an ectopic pregnancy six months ago. Investigations showed:

Hb	13 g/dl
WCC	7×10^9/l
ESR	13 mm in the first hour
CXR	Normal cardiac silhouette and fine linear opacity in the lower zone
PaO_2	7.7 kPa
$PaCO_2$	5 kPa
pH	7.5

Question

Q75.1 Suggest two possible diagnoses and their management.

Case 76

A 60-year-old Iranian refugee presented in casualty with a four-day history of fever and chest pain. He was successfully thrombolysed five months ago for a myocardial infarction and was discharged on atenolol and hydralazine for hypertension. Over the subsequent four months, he developed aches and pains in his hands, legs and back. The results of investigations showed:

Hb	12 g/dl
WCC	$5 \times 10^9/l$
Platelets	$200 \times 10^9/l$
Rheumatoid factor	Negative
ANA	Positive in 1 in 400
ECG	ST elevation in all leads
CKMB	Normal
Echo	Normal

Questions

Q76.1   What is the diagnosis?
Q76.2   What blood tests would you perform?

Case 77

A 44-year-old asthmatic accountant with a hemicolectomy scar presented to a casualty with a lobster-red face, a raised JVP, swelling of the ankles, and a pulsatile liver. He improved following emergency treatment with phenoxybenzamine. There was a palpable mass over the right hypo-chondrium. He had documented episodes of hypotension in the past, associated with increased bowel sounds and diarrhoea.

Question

Q77.1   What is the diagnosis?

Case 78

A 23-year-old interior designer, who is awaiting treatment for a mass in the neck and is on treatment for palpitations, underwent the following test following an overnight fast. She was diagnosed with possible diabetes on the basis of glycosuria. Pregnancy test was negative. The following venous blood results were obtained after a 50 g glucose load following an overnight fast:

Time (min)	Glucose (mmol/l)
0	4.6
30	12
60	5.6
90	3.2
120	4.2

Questions

Q78.1 *What is the diagnosis?*

Q78.2 *In what other conditions may this be found?*

Case 79

A 55-year-old Chilean woman, who is the chief editor of the local newspaper, suffered an anterior myocardial infarction. On her third day in the CCU, she developed further chest pain and a loud precordial friction rub. The following day, her temperature rose to 39°C and her WCC rose to 21 000/cm. Her condition improved gradually and she was discharged the next day.

In the following three weeks she felt increasingly breathless on exertion and was readmitted. A temporary pacing wire was threaded through the jugular route, as she had several episodes of hypotension associated with bradycardia. She noted a fluttering over her chest when she lay down or stooped. She then developed episodes of breathlessness with cough and sputum (but no haemoptysis). A systolic murmur was heard on the right side of the chest but she was in sinus rhythm.

Questions

Q79.1 *What are the possible diagnoses?*

Q79.2 *What investigations would you perform?*

Q79.3 *What is the prognosis?*

Q79.4 *What does the fever, pleural rub and leucocytosis suggest?*

Q79.5 *The 12-lead ECG demonstrated a RBBB pattern of pacemaker capture. What is your diagnosis?*

Case 80

A rambler who was well until the last few days developed a flu'-like illness associated with what he described as 'lumbago'. His systemic symptoms cleared after 36 hours but he complained of burning pain in both legs. Three days later, he complained of difficulty in walking and stumbled over some rocks because his vision was impaired. He was immediately admitted to hospital, where he developed urinary retention.

He had lumbar tenderness and the straight leg raising test was positive bilaterally to 20°, limited by the pain. Sensation was not affected on clinical testing although he described some paraesthesia over the left sole. Deep tendon reflexes were absent at the knee and ankles. No plantar response was elicitable. He had diplopia and there was some limitation of ocular mobility. A general physical examination appeared normal. The CXR and ECG were normal. CSF examination showed:

RBCs	25 000/mm³
Lymphocytes	10/mm³
Neutrophils	20/mm³
Glucose	6 mmol/l (with simultaneous blood glucose being 7 mmol/l)
Protein	3 g/l

Question

Q80.1 What is the diagnosis?

Case 81

A 48-year-old Sherpa underwent surgery several months ago in an isolated part of the Himalayan foothills. He made a good recovery but the original indication for the operation was never fully ascertained. He presents with chronic fatigue and malaise. A laparotomy scar was seen. Investigations showed:

Serum sodium	142 mmol/l
Serum chloride	110 mmol/l
Plasma bicarbonate	13 mmol/l
Serum potassium	3 mmol/l

Questions

Q81.1 What operation was performed?
Q81.2 What is the other explanation for this picture?

Case 82

A 22-year-old chronic asthmatic had blood taken at 8 a.m. This showed a serum cortisol of 130 nmol/l. A dose of synthetic ACTH was given i.m. and the serum cortisol half an hour later was 390 nmol/l.

Question

Q82.1 What was the diagnosis?

Case 83

A 35-year-old woman who is a membership officer of a scientific society suffered from aplastic anaemia for four years with complete recovery. Six months later at a follow-up visit the following results were obtained: antinuclear factor negative, direct antiglobulin test negative and also:

Hb	9 g/dl
Bilirubin	74 µmol/l
Urine	Contains urobilinogen and haemo-siderin
RBC cholinesterase level	Decreased
WCC	$2 \times 10^9/l$
Platelets	$90 \times 10^9/l$

A few weeks later, she had abdominal pain with increased jaundice and elevated liver enzymes.

Questions

Q83.1 What is the diagnosis?
Q83.2 What happens a few weeks later?
Q83.3 What additional investigations are required?
Q83.4 What confirms the diagnosis?
Q83.5 What would happen if you repeated the test after heating the sera?

Case 84

A 13-year-old boy who was on ventolin and slow release aminophylline, was admitted for acute breathlessness and wheezing. After treatment with nebulised salbutamol, his peak flow was still unrecordable.

Question

Q84.1 What is your subsequent management?

Case 85

A 22-year-old medical student from the Kasturba Medical College was crossing the road in Madras, when he saw the traffic stop and a crowd gathering. Walking towards the scene, he was shocked by the sight of a lorry which had crushed a young girl. She had been run over, and the intestines were pouring out from the abdomen. He felt numbed by the experience, and later discussed the statistical nature of death in a busy city, of which this is an example.

His reaction was perceived as 'cold' by his friends, who knew him to be a sensitive and dedicated idealist who was easily moved.

Questions

Q85.1 What has happened here?
Q85.2 What are the other defence mechanisms?
Q85.3 What are immature defences?
Q85.4 What are neurotic defences?
Q85.5 What are transference and countertransference?

Case 86

A 44-year-old retired police officer underwent a successful operation for a fractured hip following a car accident. His postoperative recovery appeared uneventful. Five days later, while he was having breakfast, he felt breathless at rest and complained of chest discomfort. The ECG appeared normal but a tachycardia of 100/min was noted; the CKMB level was normal. Other investigations showed:

Hb	14 g/dl
FEV_1	2.6 l (predicted 2.5–3.5)
FVC	3.6 l (predicted 3–5)
PaO_2	8 kPa
$PaCO_2$	3.1 kPa
PH	7.38

The CXR appeared normal, apart from an old healed TB scar following successfull treatment eight years ago.

Questions

Q86.1 What is the diagnosis?
Q86.2 How would you confirm this?

Q86.3 What may be seen on the CXR?
Q86.4 How would you treat this patient?

Case 87

A 55-year-old professor of anthropology fell off his roof as he tried to repair his TV aerial. An ATLS protocol was followed. His head CT scan and a CXR were normal. The peritoneal lavage was positive and all vital signs were stable. Exploratory laparotomy revealed that the spleen was ruptured and it was removed with seeding of the fragments into the peritoneum.

He made a successful postoperative recovery but developed frank painful red blotches over his skull, hands and abdomen. Investigations showed:

Hb	10 g/dl
Platelets	$20 \times 10^9/l$
PT	23 s (control of 12)
PTTK	60 s (control of 40)

There was polychromasia +++, the ECG was normal and the bowels sounds were normal.

Questions

Q87.1 What is the diagnosis?
Q87.2 How would you confirm this?
Q87.3 In what other conditions can it occur?
Q87.4 What is the treatment?

Case 88

A 21-year-old has a heart murmur since aged four. He has recently developed cyanotic attacks and dyspnoea. He has just joined the Hare Krishna movement and it was suggested that this might be a divine manifestation, as Krishna is always described as the blue God. He found it a strain to walk up stairs. He underwent cardiac catheterisation:

Site	Pressure (mmHg)	Saturation (%)
RA	7	70
RV	111/7	77
Pulmonary artery	26/11	82
Left ventricle	120/11	95

| Aorta | 120/80 | 89 |
| Left atrium | 11 | 99 |

Questions

Q88.1 What are the abnormalities?
Q88.2 What are the complications?

Case 89

A 20-year-old Bedouin had been complaining of difficulty in riding his camel and had a past history of coarctation of the aorta. He gives a two-week history of headache, nausea and vertigo. He was observed to be febrile at 38°C, with BP 140/90 mmHg, RR 26/min and a sinus rhythm of 80/min. There is a second degree nystagmus to the left, bilateral intention tremor and a left sided Babinski sign. He gives no history of excessive alcohol consumption and there is no temporal pallor of the optic disc.

Question

Q89.1 What is the diagnosis?

Case 90

A 33-year-old MSc student of manufacturing management was referred by his local psychiatrist for failing to concentrate in class. It transpired that he went 'berserk' at his wedding party three years ago. He smashed a vase outside the venue. He also gave a history of gaining weight, behaving bizarrely, falling asleep in lectures, constipation and a flaky rash. He is a regular attender of rave parties. Investigations were:

Serum calcium	2.8 mmol/l
Serum magnesium	1.1 mmol/l
ESR	1 mm in the first hour
Serum thyroxine	45 nmol/l
T_3 uptake	128%

Questions

Q90.1 What is the diagnosis and prognosis?
Q90.2 What is the acute treatment of mania?

Q90.3 *A week after discharge, he complained of headache, photo-*
phobia and vomiting. On examination, he was febrile at 39°C.
Kernig's sign was positive and neurological examination was
normal. An LP revealed the following:

Opening pressure	*18 cm water*
White cells	*220 mm (78% lymphocytes)*
Proteins	*4 g/l*
Glucose	*3 mmol/l (blood 5 mmol/l))*

He improved over the next four days. Fundoscopy revealed
papilloedema and bilateral weakness of the leg. The Babinski
reflex is bilaterally positive. What is the diagnosis?

Case 91

A 35-year-old air stewardess from Hong Kong presented with weight
loss, nausea and vomiting. She was worried that she might have
contracted "chicken 'flu". She had also noticed the growth of fine hair all
over her body and had constipation. Investigations revealed:

Plasma calcium	3 mmol/l
Plasma phosphate	0.5 mmol/l
Alkaline phosphatase	136 IU/l
Mantoux test	Negative
HIV	Negative
WCC	11 × 10⁹/l (80% neutrophils, 18% lympho cytes, 2% monocytes)
Fasting blood glucose	4 mmol/l

Question

Q91.1 What is the dignosis?

Case 92

A 66-year-old spinster was noted to have lymphadenopathy by her
friend's son who is a medical student when he was asked to comment on
shingles over her neck. She also complained of intense itching. Investigations showed:

Hb	10 g/dl
PCV	33%

MCV	82 fl
WCC	30 × 10⁹/l (30% neutrophils, 61% lymphocytes, 2% monocytes, 1% eosinophils, 3% reticulocytes)
Platelets	84 × 10⁹/l

MCV 82 fl

WCC $30 \times 10^9/l$ (30% neutrophils, 61% lymphocytes, 2% monocytes, 1% eosinophils, 3% reticulocytes)

Platelets $84 \times 10^9/l$

The peripheral blood film showed:

Spherocytes	+++
Smudge cells	+
Serum alkaline phosphatase	94 IU/l
Serum bilirubin	40 µmol/l

Question

Q92.1 What is the diagnosis?

Case 93

A retired police officer underwent a series of tests for breathlessness:

PaO_2	13.6 kPa (normal range 12–13.5)
Arterial oxygen saturation	95%
$PaCO_2$	4 kPa (normal range 4.7–6)
pH	7.4

After exercise:

PaO_2	10.4
$PaCO_2$	3.7
pH	7.56

Question

Q93.1 What is the pulmonary abnormality and how would you confirm this?

Case 94

A 55-year-old Norwegian woman complained of chronic fatigue over the past two months and had been receiving treatment for a chest infection for three months. She was complimented on an excellent sun-tan. She collapsed while waiting for a train. Investigations revealed:

Serum sodium	131 mmol/l
Serum potassium	6 mmol/l
Serum chloride	97 mmol/l
Serum bicarbonate	22 mmol/l
Blood urea	7 mmol/l

Questions

Q94.1 What is the diagnosis?
Q94.2 How should this be treated?

Case 95

A 30-year-old molecular biology postgraduate student from China complained of feeling homesick, ill and tired all the time, but was not on medication. She found herself unable to sleep at night but was drowsy and frequently dozed off during the day. She was told that it was 'the winter'. A friend told her that she might be suffering from seasonal affective disorder, and that it would improve by the spring. Her serological examination revealed:

Hb	13 g/dl
WCC	$3 \times 10^9/l$ (normal differential count)
Bilirubin	120 µmol/l
Serology for infectious mononucleosis	Negative
ALT (SGPT)	160 U/l
AST (SGOT)	400 IU/l
Serum albumin	35 g/l
HbsAg	Absent
Serum globulin	64 g/l
ANA titres	1 in 1033
Rubella and measles antibodies	High titres

Questions

Q95.1 What is the diagnosis?
Q95.2 What is the differential diagnosis of CAH?

Case 96

A 60-year-old orchestral conductor presented to casualty with chest pain, nausea and breathlessness. An inferior myocardial infarct was diagnosed. On examination his pulse was regular at 50 beats/min. The JVP was noted to be 3 cm (with a normal wave form) and the BP was 80/60. He felt dizzy on the ward, where the pulse was noted to be 45/min and regular. A stress test performed six months ago was normal.

He had felt faint while conducting a vigorous piece of Stravinski and nearly collapsed. He had had a similar feeling while having his hair washed in the barber's salon. He was on no medication at that time.

Questions

Q96.1 What is expected on the ECG and what would you advise?
Q96.2 What clinical pattern did he describe prior to this infarct?
Q96.3 In a normal anterior infarct, or in a small number of patients who become pacemaker-dependent, when should one pace and which mode is indicated?

Case 97

A 24-year-old Japanese puffer fish chef complained of weakness. Cursory examination did not suggest tetradotoxin poisoning and he had been licensed in a prestigious school in Tokyo. He appeared weak, with normal vital signs. There was no palpable cervical mass. His BP was 80/120 mmHg. He was not on penicillamine. The thyroid function tests showed that he has mild thyrotoxicosis. The results of other investigations were:

Hb	13 g/dl
PCV	40%
WCC	$6 \times 10^9/l$ (normal differential)
Sodium	140 mmol/l
Potassium	2.1 mmol/l
Bicarbonate	26 mmol/l
Renal function	Normal
ECG	No dysarrhythmia

Question

Q97.1 What is the diagnosis?

Case 98

An emaciated-looking 45-year-old Japanese man who works in an automobile plant complained of a dull abdominal ache, loss of appetite for the last three months and weight loss. He is on antihypertensive therapy and is taking oral antacids. Investigations showed:

Blood urea	15 mmol/l
Plasma sodium	134 mmol/l
Plasma potassium	3.2 mmol/l

Questions

Q98.1 What is the diagnosis?
Q98.2 What will be the pH of the urine?
Q98.3 Why has this patient got metabolic alkalosis?

Case 99

A 46-year-old Aikido instructor became progressively breathless and unable to complete his kata. Investigations revealed heart failure. His wife described impotence and polyuria as some of his problems. On investigation:

Hb	14 g/dl
PCV	52%
WCC	10 × 10⁹/l (83% neutrophils)
Fasting blood glucose	12 mmol/l
Serum albumin	40 g/l
Serum ALT (SGPT)	132 IU/l
Serum iron	64 µmol/l
Iron binding capacity	71 µmol/l

Questions

Q99.1 What is the diagnosis?
Q99.2 How else may this condition present?
Q99.3 How should this patient be treated?

Case 100

An eccentric, thin 76-year-old man, who grows all his own marijuana and survives on canned food, pulses and new-age food, was being investigated for bruising (diagnosed as senile purpura). He complained of back pain and breast enlargement. The Hess test is strongly positive. There is no history of recent travel abroad. Investigations showed:

PT   13 s (control 13 s)
PTTK   50 s (control 37 s)
Platelets 200×10^9/l

Questions

Q100.1 What is the diagnosis?

Q100.2 What else should be assessed?

Q100.3 One week after hospitalisation he demonstrated a relatively normal PT but a prolonged PTT. What has happened?

Case 101

A 33-year-old Jesuit priest developed severe breathlessness. He has been taking medication for a peptic ulcer. Arterial blood gas determination showed a PaO_2 of 7 kPa and a $PaCO_2$ of 4.3 kPa.

Question

Q101.1 What are the possible diagnoses?

Case 102

A 56-year-old mathematics teacher collapsed after bending to pick up a piece of chalk in a calculus class. She gave a history of dysphagia for the last five years due to chronic reflux oesophagitis. She recovered on admission to casualty but felt nauseous and sweated profusely. She felt dizzy and had to be supported when she tried to get up. On examination, she was noted to have long spidery fingers and both her plantar responses were extensor (Babinski positive). Her BP was 90/60 mmHg and Hb was 12 g/dl.

Questions

Q102.1 What is the diagnosis?

Q102.2 How would you diagnose it?

Case 103

A 45-year-old Romanian army officer has been complaining for two months of breathlessness and palpitations. He has been treated for bronchial airway hyperreactivity. He had no health problems according to a cursory recruitment check-up 20 years ago. On examination, he had a regular pulse of 90 per minute, the JVP was raised with a prominent 'a' wave, and auscultation revealed a 'sail like sound' at the left sternal border. ECG shows a RBBB, a broad QRS complex with a slurring upstroke, very large P waves which appear bifid, right axis deviation and a PR interval of three small squares. The CXR shows a large heart. He was noted to be mildly cyanosed.

Questions

Q103.1 What is the diagnosis and how will you confirm this?
Q103.2 How would you treat the palpitations?

Case 104

A 43-year-old nuclear physicist, who works out regularly at the gym, presents with a headache and a 'sense of being lost at sea at times'. He won the Weider bodybuilding competition last year and had been taking anabolic steroids. When his supply 'dried up' because of police vigilance, he started obtaining growth hormones illicitly from Hungary. He also rides horses on a competitive basis.

He was making mistakes in rudimentary calculations and had been uncharacteristically ill-tempered for the last three weeks. He complained of epsodic 'twitching movements over his pectoral muscles'and became lost in a security facility in which he had been working for the last four years. He has been uncharacteristically 'clumsy'. The CT scan and CSF examination were normal and he is HIV negative. A routine drug screen and VDRL were negative. TFTs and the B_{12} level were normal. The EEG showed periodic biphasic high-amplitude sharp waves.

Questions

Q104.1 What is the most likely diagnosis?
Q104.2 What is the gold standard for the diagnosis of this disease?

Case 105

An 18-year-old A-level science student complained of amenorrhoea. There was no history of any weight loss. She had been referred to a dental surgeon for assessment of badly eroded teeth. Her parotid glands were enlarged. On examination, she had scratch marks over the dorsum of the second knuckle. Clinical examination was otherwise normal. She runs five miles daily, rain or shine. The results of investigations were:

Plasma sodium	136 mmol/l
Plasma potassium	2.8 mmol/l
Serum urea	5 mmol/l
Blood film	Normal

Questions

Q105.1 What is the diagnosis?
Q105.2 What other states may present with such a biochemical profile?

Case 106

A 25-year-old model who is taking pills made of seal liver extract and other herbs complained to her GP of headache, irritability, loss of hair, and has dry and scaly skin. She has noticed progressive blurring of vision. On examination, she was afebrile and there is papilloedema. Other findings include hepatomegaly and palpation of the tip of the spleen. All other systems appear normal. Routine electrolyte and biochemical profiles appear normal.

Question

Q106.1 What is the diagnosis?

Case 107

A 35-year-old art teacher who underwent a late abortion for foetal abnormalities detected by amniocentesis five days ago was readmitted for vaginal bleeding. She was febrile at 38.5°C, there was a tachycardia of 180/min and the uterus appeared to have involuted normally. On admission she fitted violently and lapsed into a coma. The blood sugar level estimated at that time was normal and no neurological localising sounds were found. Initial investigations showed:

Hb	4 g/dl
WCC	15×10^9/l
Platelets	12×10^9/l
Blood film	Occasional contracted cells and spherocytes
DAGT	Negative
Clotting screen	Normal
FDPs	Normal

Serum urea   35 mmol/l
Serum creatinine   315 µmol/l

Questions

Q107.1 What is the likely diagnosis?
Q107.2 What is the treatment?

Case 108

A 23-year-old homeless mainliner (injecting heroin from a Detroit supplier), who begs for a living, presented with a two-month history of night sweats and a recent unproductive cough. There was no history of cardiac disease. On examination, he had oral candidiasis, oral petechiae, a staring mask-like face, and signs of rigidity and bradykinesia. He was febrile at 38.5°C and auscultation revealed bilateral basal crackles. Investigations showed:

Hb   12 g/dl
WCC $4 \times 10^9/l$
CXR   Normal

Arterial blood gas pressures in air were:

PaO_2 9 kPa
$PaCO_2$ 4 kPa

Questions

Q108.1 What is the diagnosis and how should this be managed?
Q108.2 Why is he so rigid?
Q108.3 A few months after starting antiretroviral therapy, he com-
plained of shooting pains and weakness on climbing stairs.
Investigations showed: Hb 8 g/l, WCC 3 × $10^9/l$, Platelets 100 ×
$10^9/l$, MCV 94 fl and CPK 655 IU/l. What is the diagnosis?

Case 109

A 25-year-old female pianist is described as 'weird' by her friends and has started going out with a new boyfriend. She has a past history of convulsions and had problems with sleeping, so her boyfriend gave her a barbiturate which he had bought while on holiday in Mexico. Over the next few days she started complaining of severe abdominal pain, but a home pregnancy test kit showed that she was not pregnant. She became irritable and was unable to play the piano because she felt her fingers to be dead.

Clinical examination revealed a laparotomy scar, which the files described as no pathology detected. There was no organomegaly. She had signs of dorsiflexion of the left wrist and a VI cranial nerve palsy of the right eye. Fundoscopy was normal and she gave no history suggestive of lead exposure. During the interview with the physician, she suddenly turned round to a blank wall and shouted, 'And the same to you too!'

Questions

Q109.1 What is the diagnosis?
Q109.2 How would you confirm the diagnosis?
Q109.3 How would you manage her?

Case 110

A 28-year-old jazz musician had just returned from a trip to New Orleans. He has a past history of a heart murmur for which he was given a 'guarded' prognosis. He lived each day, cherishing it as his last. He underwent cardiac catheterisation as he had turned blue and developed clubbing:

Chamber	Oxygen saturation (%)
RA	66
RV	64
Pulmonary artery	70
LA	88
LV	75
Aorta	79

Question

Q110.1 What is the diagnosis?

Case 111

A 26-year-old air hostess gave a 4-month history of periodic disorientation, blurred vision, light headedness, and palpitations accompanied by profuse sweating. She has been gaining weight and nearly fainted twice while serving duty-free goods. Her son is a diabetic. Investigations showed:

Hb	13 g/dl
WCC	5 × 10⁹/l
Serum sodium	138 mmol/l
Serum potassium	4.3 mmol/l
Serum urea	4 mmol/l
LFT	normal

Random blood glucose measured when the patient was symptomatic was 3 mmol/l. After a 12-hour fast (during symptoms):

Blood glucose	1.5 mmol/l
Insulin	55 mU/l
Insulin:glucose ratio	36.6 (normal range < 10)

Questions

Q111.1 What is the diagnosis?
Q111.2 What investigations would you perform?
Q111.3 What is the definitive treatment?

Case 112

A 60-year-old stoic Caribbean woman who has felt ill for weeks has been taking Lucozade for 'flu'. She gave a four-day history of dysuria and urinary frequency. On examination, she was pyrexial (38.5°C) drowsy, disorientated and severely dehydrated. The investigation results were:

Hb	16 g/dl
WCC	20 × 10⁹/l (90% neutrophils)
Plasma sodium	130 mmol/l
Plasma potassium	5.3 mmol/l
Plasma chloride	128 mmol/l
Plasma bicarbonate	22 mom/l
Plasma urea	32 mmol/l

Urinalysis showed pus cells ++++ and glucose 5+G. Ketones were negative.

Questions

Q112.1 What is the likely diagnosis?
Q112.2 What are the essential investigations?
Q112.3 How would you treat this condition?
Q112.4 How would you analyse hyponatraemia?

Case 113

A 45-year-old Peruvian man who is being treated for miliary TB had the following blood results:

Hb	10 g/dl
PCV	38%
MCHC	29 g/dl
WCC	13 × 10⁹/l (63% neutrophils, 28% lymphocytes, 3% monocytes, 4% metamyelocytes and 2% myelocytes)

There were nucleated RBCs and relatively few platelets.

Questions

Q113.1 What has occurred?
Q113.2 How is this confirmed?
Q113.3 What other conditions may cause this?

Case 114

A struggling artist who helps the local publican in exchange for food and lodging in the attic, was admitted to hospital because of a worsening cough, dyspnoea and 'flu-like symptoms each winter for the last two years. There were no budgerigars in the house. The CXR showed fine miliary infiltration. Investigations showed:

FEV$_1$	3 litres
FVC	3.5 litres
DCO (TCO)	9 ml min^{-1} (predicted at 24 ml min^{-1} mmHg^{-1})
PaO$_2$	10 kPa
PaCO$_2$	3 kPa

Questions

Q114.1 What is the diagnosis?

Q114.2 *What pattern of lung function abnormalities may be deduced?*
Q114.3 *What is the treatment?*
Q114.4 *How do you analyse interstitial lung disease (ILD)?*

Case 115

A 35-year-old Cuban refugee who is taking carbamazepine for tri-geminal neuralgia, was admitted for a convulsive episode. He gives a history of several fits in the past two months and says he had not been feeling himself. He started fitting again while being examined. The blood film was normal:

Hb	14 g/dl
WCC	10×10^9/l
Platelets	160×10^9/l
Serum creatinine	80 mmol/l
Serum sodium	124 mmol/l
Serum potassium	4 mmol/l
Serum glucose	5 mmol/l
Serum lipids	Normal
Brain CT	Normal
TFT	Normal

Questions

Q115.1 *What is the diagnosis?*
Q115.2 *What is the treatment?*

Case 116

A 33-year-old accountant who had been treated for years for hyper-tension, left for a 'holiday' in the Cayman islands. Two days after landing, he attended casualty complaining of severe insomnia, headache, sweating and agitation. On examination, he had a tachycardia of 110/min and SR with occasional ectopics. The ECG did not show changes suggestive of an infarct or ischaemia; the BP was 220/150 mmHg. He was admitted and the urinary catecholamine excre-tion was 17 μmol over 24 hours.

Questions

Q116.1 *What is the differential diagnosis?*
Q116.2 *How should he be treated?*

Case 117

A 35-year-old woman presented with weakness. She had marital problems as a result of keeping her husband awake all night because she has nocturia. He complains that she goes to the toilet six times a night. She was found to be hypertensive at 177/110 mmHg and fundoscopy showed AV nipping. There was no renal bruit. Investigations showed:

Serum sodium	143 mmol/l
Serum potassium	3.3 mmol/l
Serum bicarbonate	29 mmol/l
Serum urea	5 mmol/l

After a normal saline infusion over six hours, it was noted that her BP was still high but the serum sodium was 146 mmol/l and the serum potassium 3.1 mmol/l.

Questions

Q117.1 What is the diagnosis?

Q117.2 What are the other causes of polyuria?

Case 118

A 14-year-old ballet student was worried that she might not grow tall enough to be a professional dancer. She was investigated and noted to be shorter than her peers. There was no familial history of delayed developmental growth or delayed menarche. On examination, there appeared to be an absence of pubertal development. A combined anterior pituitary function test was performed with insulin 0.15 µg/kg i.v., TRH 200 µg i.v. and LHRH 100 µg i.v.:

Time (min)	Glucose (mmol/l)	Cortisol (nmol/l)	GH (mU/l)	TSH (mU/l)	LH (IU/l)	FSH (IU/l)
0	5	360	< 1	2	> 25	> 50
15	2	400	17	–	–	–
30	9	450	25	12	> 25	> 50
45	2.8	670	15	–	–	–
60	3.9	584	8	7	> 25	> 50
90	4	474	5	–	–	–

Questions

Q118.1 What is the diagnosis? ✓
Q118.2 How is this confirmed? ✓

Case 119

An 8-year-old child with multiple bruises and a recent onset of epistaxis was reviewed by a consultant who identified the marks on the buttocks as Mongolian spots and not child abuse. The haematological indices were reported as:

Hb	8 g/dl
WCC	7×10^9/l
Platelets	200×10^9/l
Reticulocytes	5%
Bleeding time	32 min
PT	13 s (control 13 s)
PTT	60 s (control 45 s)
Factor VIII level	19%

Questions

Q119.1 What is the most likely diagnosis?
Q119.2 What is the abnormality in this disorder?
Q119.3 How would you treat this disorder?

Case 120

A 35-year-old bungee jumping enthusiast presented to clinic with progressive shortness of breath. He has a family history of respiratory disease. His pulmonary function results were as follows:

FEV$_1$	1.1 litre (3.7)
FVC	3.0 litre (4.2)
TLC	7.0 litre (5.1)
TF	11 litre (28)

Questions

Q120.1 What is the diagnosis? ✓
Q120.2 What are the genetic variations of this disorder?
Q120.3 What other clinical manifestations may this patient have?

Case 121

A 44-year-old Jamaican trader celebrated a successful deal with an oriental dish of Dover sole and wine, but suddenly felt nauseous and retched. He gave no history suggestive of allergy to monosodium glutamate. He collapsed and was admitted to casualty shocked, breathless and describing an excruciating pain in the chest. The ECG and immediate CKMB, serum amylase and electrolyte levels were all normal. The CXR showed a left pleural effusion and air in the mediastinum.

Questions

Q121.1 What is the diagnosis? ✓
Q121.2 What is the therapy? ✓
Q121.3 What is a 'café' coronary? ✓

Case 122

A 55-year-old man who was on therapy for relapsing polychondritis was a regular participant in the MRCP clinical examination. He complained that he needed more pillows to prop him up at night. He also gave a history suggestive of severe PND. Cardiac catheterisation demonstrated:

	Pressure (mmHg)	
	Phasic	Mean
RA	–	6
RV	60/0–8	–
Pulmonary artery	45–55/20	30
Wedge	–	30
LV	145/19–24	–
LVEDP	18–22	–
Aorta	145/40	–

Questions

Q122.1 What is the diagnosis? ✓
Q122.2 When should one operate in endocarditis? ✓

Case 123

A 44-year-old milkman, who had recently divorced, complained of itching in his eyes. He was reviewed in the clinic with the following investigation results:

Serum creatinine	125 μmol/l
Liver function tests	Normal
Serum alkaline phosphatase	Normal
Total serum protein	50 g/l
Serum albumin	29 g/l
Serum urate	0.7 mmol/l
Serum calcium	3 mmol/l
Serum phosphate	1.2 mmol/l
Serum cholesterol	9 mmol/l
Serum triglycerides	2 mmol/l

Questions

Q123.1 What is the diagnosis?
Q123.2 How would you confirm this?
Q123.3 What is the prognosis?
Q123.4 What are the bad prognostic indicators of myeloma?

Case 124

A 30-year-old sales manager of a Fortune 500 company, who has recently joined Weight Watchers for obesity, complains of acne (for which she is taking Roaccutane). She complains of irregular menstruation and lethargy, and was admitted to be investigated. The results were:

Hb	18 g/dl
PCV	0.6%
Plasma potassium	3 mmol/l
Plasma bicarbonate	32 mmol/l

The results of an OGTT (75 g) were:

Time (min)	Glucose (mmol/l)
0	5
30	17
120	14

Questions

Q124.1 What is the diagnosis?

Q124.2 What investigations would you perform?

Q124.3 What is a flat glucose tolerance curve?

Case 125

A 50-year-old zoo keeper, who is on long-term therapy for a chest problem, presented with the following haematological indices:

Hb	8 g/dl
MCV	97 fl
Reticulocytes	1.4%
Platelets	$110 \times 10^9/l$
WCC	$8 \times 10^9/l$ (55% neutrophils, 35% lymphocytes, 65% monocytes, 2% eosinophils and 2% basophils)

The blood film showed a dimorphic blood picture.

Questions

Q125.1 What is the diagnosis?

Q125.2 How would you classify this disorder?

Case 126

A 45-year-old wealthy stockbroker has been feeling unwell for the last three weeks and described several episodes suggestive of melaena but he is also taking iron supplements. He has been described as paranoid by his wife whom he believes is having an affair with a lawyer. He claimed that she asked him to change his will recently and that her previous husbands had died in mysterious circumstances. He met her through a lonely hearts column. He has ordered some remote surveillance equipment and told his psychologist that he believes that his wife is poisoning him. He was diagnosed by the therapist as suffering from systematic delusion and that he has a borderline personality disorder. In the meantime, his results revealed:

Hb	14 g/dl
Platelets	$250 \times 10^9/l$
Bleeding time	5 min
PT	70 s (normal range up to 15 s)
PTT	56 (normal 40 s)
TT	13 s (normal 13 s)

Questions

Q126.1 **What is the diagnosis?**

Case 127

A 24-year-old Israeli archaeology student complains of typical precordial discomfort which radiates to the left arm while he watches TV. He appears normal on clinical examination and echocardiography. He has a normal exercise stress test and a routine blood test reveals a triglyceride level of 2.8 mmol/l and a serum cholesterol of 11 mmol/l.

Questions

Q127.1 **What is the diagnosis?**
Q127.2 **What treatment should be advised?**
Q127.3 **What other test may you perform?**
Q127.4 **What if he complained of a band-like pain over the left side of his chest, haematuria and impotence?**

Case 128

A 10-year-old schoolboy was admitted for assessment of precocious sexual development. At the age of four years, he was noted by the parents to have developed pubic hair. He also grew much taller than expected and the shaft of his penis grew beyond the norm of his peers. There were acrimonious arguments after his birth because the population in the small village in which they lived felt that he was not of the same race, and his mother was ostracised. On examination, he appeared muscular and had a dark, greasy skin. Axillary and pubic hairs were noted and the penile size corresponded with his pubertal development. All other systems examination were normal. The results of investigations were:

Hb	12 g/dl
WCC	7×10^9/l
ESR	4 mm/h
Serum urea	4 mmol/l
Serum sodium	135 mmol/l
Serum potassium	5 mmol/l
Serum bicarbonate	20 mmol/l
Serum chloride	106 mmol/l
Serum bilirubin	15 mmol/l

Serum alkaline phosphatase	200 mmol/l
Total protein	63 g/l
Serum calcium	2.3 mmol/l
Serum phosphate	199 mmol/l
Plasma renin level	7000 pmol/l (normal range 230–1000 pmol/l)
Bone age	12 years

Questions

Q128.1 What is the most likely diagnosis?
Q128.2 How would you confirm it?

Case 129

A 38-year-old Rabbi presented with dyspepsia and vague aches all over his body. He noticed that he was passing black stools (although he was not taking iron tablets). He felt that he was losing his faith. The investigations showed a Hb level of 10 g/l and the film was microcytic and hypochromic. The results of other investigations were:

Blood urea	5 mmol/l
Serum albumin	40 mmol/l
Serum magnesium	1.3 mmol/l
Serum phosphate	0.8 mmol/l
Serum alkaline phosphatase	60 IU/l
Serum urate	0.3 mmol/day
Urine calcium excretion	8 mmol/day
Urine culture	*E. coli*

Questions

Q129.1 What is the diagnosis?
Q129.2 How would you confirm and treat this disease?

Case 130

A gypsy couple found that they woke up feeling drowsy and forgetful during mid-winter. The wife reported an episode of convulsions a few days ago. They live in an old but well-heated caravan. They were brought to casualty in a comatose state this morning. There were no needle marks and a thorough search did not reveal any illicit drugs.

Questions

Q130.1 What is the diagnosis? ✓
Q130.2 What is the treatment? ✓

Case 131

A 23-year-old Irish missionary, who lives at the edge of the Amazon forest, has been told that he has had a heart murmur since he was a child. No further tests were done as he seems well and able to cope with the rigors of tropical parish life. He has also raised two children. Investigations showed:

	Pressure (mmHg)	O_2 saturation (%)
SVC	67	
RA	3	68
Low RV	62/5	69
High RV	62/5	74
Pulmonary artery	63/24	84
Femoral artery	94/74	95

Question

Q131.1 What is the initial diagnosis? ✓

Case 132

A 55-year-old sergeant, who has smoked two packs of cigarettes a day for the last 20 years, complained of cough and breathlessness for two weeks. He had noticed clumsiness of his arms and was thought to be drunk despite being teetotal. The preliminary blood reports were:

Serum sodium	130 mmol/l
Serum chloride	84 mmol/l
Serum potassium	3 mmol/l
Serum calcium	3.2 mmol/l

He is worried that he may have TB as one of the soldiers he trained was recently diagnosed with this condition. The CT scan showed cerebellar degeneration but no focal lesions.

Question

Q132.1 What is the diagnosis? ✓

Case 133

A diver operating off the coast of Borneo had trained himself to spend five minutes with no air under water. He dives regularly to forage for oysters and repeatedly pushes himself to the surface gasping for air and handing over the spoils of his search to his wife. On one occasion, he guided a group of tourists up to a hill resort after diving. He suddenly felt breathless after paralysing a wildfowl with his blowpipe. He also experienced urinary problems, pain and numbness in all his muscles, and behaved strangely, shouting expletives at his tour group. Rashes appeared over his abdomen and he suddenly collapsed.

Questions

Q133.1 What is the diagnosis? ✓
Q133.2 If they had eaten the wildfowl, what complications would there have been? ✓

Case 134

A 27-year-old Iranian virologist presented with a three-year history of progressive breathlessness on exertion, in association with chest pain and fatigue. She collapsed while climbing a flight of stairs at the airport. She has also noticed her voice becoming more hoarse and she gave a history of one episode of haemoptysis and being treated for schistosomiasis.

Clinical examination revealed that she was tachypnoeic at rest, afebrile and had nicotine-stained fingers. The JVP was recorded as 7 cm and prominent 'a' waves were observed. There is a left parasternal heave and a palpable P2. There was a normal first heart sound and a loud P_2, which 'split' normally. There was also a soft mid-diastolic murmur, loudest during inspiration. The CXR was normal. The ECG showed a tall 'p' wave in lead II. There was a tall R wave and inverted T waves in leads V1, V2 and V3.

Questions

Q134.1 What is the diagnosis? ✓
Q134.2 What are the causes of this disorder? ✓
Q134.3 How would you investigate her? ✓

Case 135

A 42-year-old paediatrician complained of pain in both ears and pharyngitis since arriving in Hong Kong three weeks ago. She had returned from London to watch the historical raising of the Chinese flag, which was a prerequisite for retaining her right of abode in the former colony. She had no relatives and found the hotels all booked, so had to live with an acquaintance. She complained of loose stools with no blood, which she attributed to the food. On examination, she was febrile with a temperature of 38.5°C. Her pulse was 110/min and regular, the BP normal and the results of biochemical tests revealed:

Hep B	Negative
T_4	38 nmol/l (normal range 10–26)
FT_3	8 pmol/l (normal range 3–8)
ANA	Negative
Thyroid autoantibodies	Negative
TSH	< 0.1 (normal range 0.4–6.0)

Questions

Q135.1 What is the diagnosis?
Q135.2 How is it diagnosed?
Q135.3 How would you treat her?

Answers

Case 1

Q1.1   What is the diagnosis?

Answer 1.1

The antihistamine predisposed this gentleman to heat stroke, with cardiac failure due to increased pulmonary output in this state. This is not uncommon for those travelling by jet to the equator during winter. Heat strokes were reported in Vietnam in association with amphetamines. Other predisposing causes include tricyclic antidepressants, phenothiazines, cord trauma and cystic fibrosis.

Therapy involves cooling the patient aggressively with cold water, i.v. glucose infusion and monitoring the serum potassium level. Heat stroke is common in pilgrims travelling to Mecca and therefore they should be adequately informed before embarking on such a journey. The Saudi Arabian protocol includes the use of ice externally, fans, and nasogastric infusion of cool fluids.

The presence of petechiae must evoke the possibility of dengue fever, which is not uncommon in this region. Therapy for dengue fever is generally supportive. Malaria is another possibility but the absence of a palpable spleen suggests that this is not the case. However, this must be ruled out by a thick and thin blood film, carried out on three separate occasions.

The complications of malaria are hypoglycaemia, which may be quinine induced, renal failure, splenic rupture and DIC.

Q1.2   How would you treat this patient if he had presented with the same symptoms in England?

Answer 1.2

Intravenous penicillin or ceftriaxome should be given immediately as the mortality of early undiagnosed meningococcal meningitis is high, and one should err on the side of caution. If meningococcal meningitis is confirmed, closed contacts should be given prophylactic rifampicin.

Q1.3   How would you approach this patient if his CK is above 1000 IU/l, his urine is black and the dipstick is positive?

Answer 1.3

This is highly suggestive of rhabdomyolysis. The dipstick is positive for blood and myoglobin. An immediate microscopic examination of the urine would show myoglobin. Cases of marathon runners suffering from rhabdomyolysis, liver necrosis, acute tubular necrosis of the kidney, pulmonary aspiration, seizures and coma have been reported in the young. Cases of rhabdomyolysis have been reported in firemen during intensive drill.

The mainstay of therapy should be hydration. A CVP line should be inserted to ensure that one is not overloading the patient. The Israeli crush injury trials suggest that early alkalinisation of the urine may prevent myoglobinuric kidneys. Dialysis should be performed if the patient becomes hyperkalaemic. Hyperkalaemia *per se* is toxic to the kidney. The causes of death in rhabdomyolysis are acidosis, renal failure, DIC and hyperkalaemia. These complications should be anticipated and treated in the acute phase.

Q1.4   *He was discharged from hospital on erythromycin, for presumed chest infection, and terfenadine. The ECG showed a QRS duration of 0.4 s on discharge. He died on the tarmac of the airport. What had happened?*

Answer 1.4

The lethal combination of these two drugs predisposed the patient to *torsades de pointes*.

Case 2

Q2.1   *What is the likely diagnosis?*

A2.1

The faecal fat is malabsorbed but the D-xylose excretion is normal, suggesting chronic pancreatitis. It is difficult to separate acute from chronic pancreatitis but it has been agreed that alcohol may cause the first attack acutely. It is rare for acute pancreatitis to occur in the absence of pain. Steatorrhoea (which may be assessed by the Lundh test meal for assessment of the exocrine function) occurs when secretion of pancreatic lipase drops below 90%.

The fainting spells are due to hypoglycaemic attacks as there is a deficiency of glucagon. The pancreolaureal test is a possible alternative non-invasive test of pancreatic function, using flourescein dilaurate and measuring its excretion in the urine as a timed sample.

Q2.2   *What are the possible underlying causes of this condition?*

A2.2

His age and occupation suggests chronic alcohol consumption. Another possibility not to be missed is a pancreatic neoplasm if the history is short. It is important not to miss the significance of the raised amylase when treating hypercalcaemia due to cancer.

Q2.3   Suggest some useful investigations.

A2.3

Abdominal X-ray examination may show calcification (or ileus in the acute stage). If the serum amylase is elevated five times above normal, the diagnosis of acute pancreatitis is very likely. A CT scan and ultrasonography may demonstrate distortion of the pancreatic duct, or detect the 'culprit' stone. The development of diabetes is common. ERCP may be helpful once the patient is stabilised. Catheterisation of the splenic artery is performed in some centres.

Supplementary Question 2.4   What if he develops an abdominal mass after 10 days with fever?

Supplementary Answer A2.4

One must diagnose a pancreatic abscess or a phlegmon. A pancreatic abscess is the secondary infection of a peripancreatic collection of fluid. There is a raised WCC and persistent fever. This clinical deterioration may be associated with ARDS, and cardiac and renal problems.

Supplementary Question 2.5   How do you demonstrate steatorrhoea by the breath test?

Supplementary Answer A2.5

By comparing the amount of exhaled $^{14}CO_2$ following the ingestion of labelled fatty acid (e.g. oleic acid) with that following the ingestion of labelled triglyceride (e.g. triolein), one may compare ^{14}C oleic acid with ^{14}C triolein. A drop in triglyceride absorption with normal fatty acid absorption indicates pancreatic dysfunction.

Supplementary Question 2.6   Is it possible to have acute pancreatitis with a normal serum amylase?

Supplementary Answer A2.6

This is rare but possible. After multiple episodes of pancreatitis, there would be insufficient pancreatic tissue to raise the amylase level during an acute attack, but the lipase level may rise. Another cause is hyperlipidaemia type IV, which interferes with amylase assays. Late assays may miss the peak serum level.

Supplementary Question Q2.7   What are the most reliable prognostic indicators in patients with acute pancreatitis?

Supplementary Answer A2.7

Glucose	$> 10\,mmol/l$
Calcium	$< 2\,mmol/l$
Urea	$> 16\,mmol/l$
PaO_2	$< 7.5\,kPa$
AST	$> 100\,IU/l$
WCC	$> 16 \times 10^9/l$

Case 3

Q3.1 What is the significance of the stress test?

A3.1

Hippocrates first described the importance of knowing the common diseases prevalent in a geographical zone as an aid to the accuracy of diagnosis. This was later scientifically described by Bayes' theorem. A fit young female athlete with a positive stress test has a low probability of significant coronary atheroma unless there is a history of familial hypercholesterolaemia. The past history of an infarct increases the likelihood in the above patient. It is important not to repeat the dependent variables in calculating the probability of a test.

Syndrome X is a positive stress test with normal coronary arteries (where paradoxically this cohort tends to live longer than their pain-free counterparts). A stress test in England will have a specificity of 85% and a sensitivity of 60% in a man such as described above.

A failing ventricle is indicated by failure of the arterial pressure to rise under stress but the best indicator of myocardial reserve is the ability to walk on the flat for at least a mile. A normal response is shown by a progressive BP rise with an increase in workload.

Q3.2 When should one perform a coronary angiogram?

A3.2

Coronary angiography should be performed only if one plans to revascularise the patient. CABG should be performed in those with significant stenosis of the left main stem or three-vessel disease.

Q3.3 What is the difference between sensitivity and specificity of a test?

A3.3

The sensitivity is the probability of identifying correctly a case of disease. It is synonymous with a 'true positive rate'. The formula for sensitivity is true positives divided by (true positives + false negatives).

On the other hand, the specificity is the probability of identifying correctly a non-diseased person who had been screened as 'false positive'. The formula for specificity is true negatives divided by (true negatives + false positives).

The positive predictive value of the test is the probability that a person receiving the positive result has the disease. This is calculated as true positives divided by (true positives + false positives).

Q3.4   What is the difference between a type I and a type II error?

A3.4

A type I error is a rejection of the null hypothesis when it is true. This is an error of commission. An analogy of a type I error may be the fabrication of clinical signs where there are none. This is highly dangerous as a patient may be diagnosed on clinical grounds to have ankylosing spondylitis and started on therapy when he has Forestier's disease. This is not as improbable as one would imagine. Most people with ankylosing spondylitis have HLA B27 but not all people with HLA B27 have ankylosing spondylitis.

A type II error is a failure to reject the null hypothesis when it is false. This is an error of omission. A crude analogy of a type II error would be to reject the hypothesis that crossing a road is hazardous. This may translate false security when it is, in fact, hazardous.

The null hypothesis is the assumption that the findings are by chance.

Q3.5   What is syndrome X pertaining to insulin resistance?

A3.5

This is the combination of hyperinsulinaemia in association with obesity, glucose intolerance, hypertension and dyslipoproteinaemia. It is associated with patients with NIDDM and the obesity is characteristically central in nature. The lipid abnormalities are characterised by an increased VLDL and a reduced HDL. It is associated with a high risk for coronary artery disease.

Case 4

Q4.1   What is the diagnosis?

A4.1

Rhombencephalitis. The brain stem signs are characteristic of *Listeria monocytogenes*. This infection is usually seen in neonates, pregnant women and the immunocompromised.

Q4.2   What investigations would you pursue?

A4.2

Diagnosis is by a history of cheese or delicatessen food intake. Culture by cold enrichment is easier from blood than from CSF. The immune status of the patient should be assessed.

Q4.3   What is the therapy?

A4.3

Listeria is sensitive to i.v. ampicillin in high doses.

Case 5

Q5.1   What are the possible diagnoses?

A5.1

This is vitamin D deficiency, either because of dietary insufficiency or malabsorption. This is the clinical presentation of rickets. Pseudo-fractures were first noted by Caffey and still carry his name. They are incomplete lines of periosteal erosion over the long bones or the scapula (also called the milkman's fracture). The clinical profile is in keeping with the child's deficiency and there may be bowing of the legs, deformity of the skull and a rickety rosary, which consists of swellings over the costochondral junction. The markings on his buttocks are Mongolian blue spots, which are birthmarks.

Case 6

Q6.1   What is the significance of these results and why did he develop nocturia?

A6.1

This points to the diagnosis of diabetes insipidus as he lost 4 kg of fluids in eight hours, yet the kidneys had not increased their capacity to concentrate the urine. This reflects, a lack of ADH. A normal response of fluid deprivation for eight hours is a weight loss of less than 0.5 kg body weight and a rise in urinary osmolality of 700–1000 mosmol/kg otherwise *Homo sapiens* would not have been able to populate the widely dispersed Polynesian islands or traverse the African deserts.

This man literally has no anterior pituitary. Cortisol increased his ability to lose water (which is physiologically normal) to the point of nocturia. This is known as the 'permissive' action of cortisol. In addition to anterior pituitary failure, he has posterior pituitary failure, which was masked by cortisol deficiency.

Case 7

Q7.1   What are the possible diagnoses and how would you investigate?

A7.1

Thalassaemia major (which may be a genetic legacy from the Armada) and pyridoxine responsive anaemia are the possibilities. An empirical trial of pyridoxine will unveil this, and electrophoresis will demonstrate thalassaemia. One must also consider sideroblastic anaemia (thus a history of lead pica and antituberculous therapy is vital). The characteristic bony changes in thalassaemia major are due to peripheral marrow attempts to produce defective RBCs resulting in the squirrel face and the hair-on-end appearance (and on X-ray). The short bones of the hands are rectangular with a trabeculated medulla giving a mosaic pattern. In the long bones, the cortices are thinned and the medulla is thickened and visible on X-ray.

Q7.2   What is the management of this disorder?

A7.2

The aim is to prevent ineffective erythropoiesis by regular iron repletion. This may damage the heart (which should be regularly monitored by echocardiography and ECG) and other vital organs. Haemosiderosis may be prevented by monitoring the serum transferrin.

Bone marrow transplantation has an 80% success rate in HLA typed siblings but there is a 10% mortality due to graft versus host reaction. With this treatment, the patient achieves puberty and normal sexual development, but compliance may be a problem. Desferrioxamine with ascorbic acid (which increases the rate of iron secretion) reduces the iron overload. Desferrioxamine can cause cataracts, deafness and retinopathy. Patients on this chelator are prone to *Yersinia enterocolitica*. If the iron requirement escalates rapidly, one may perform a splenectomy but it is best to wait until the patient is six years old to reduce the risk of infection with encapsulated organisms, after which, prophylaxis is required. The electrophoresis shows a high HbF, and low MCV and MCH, which simulates iron deficiency anaemia.

Genetic counselling should also be offered to all patients and family members.

Case 8

Q8.1   *Has the child got syphilis?*

A8.1

Yes, as IgM is too big to pass the placenta.

Case 9

Q9.1   *What has happened to the creatinine clearance?*

A9.1

Using the formula *UV/P*, where *U* is the urinary excretion of creatinine, *V* the volume of urine per minute and *P* the plasma creatinine concentration, the calculated creatinine clearance is above normal. This may be seen in proteinuria as excess creatinine is lost in the urine. It is also possible that the lowered albumin level allows increased quantities of creatinine to pass the glomerulus.

In the early stages of diabetic nephropathy, it is possible to retard the progression to ESRD by the early use of an ACE inhibitor as it reduces the intraglomerular hydrostatic trauma when microalbuminuria is first detected.

Renal failure reduces the insulin requirement.

Q9.2   *This man presents 20 years later because of 'fatigue' and has not been complying well with the treatment prescribed. He is confused and has noticed occasional 'twitching' of his pectoral muscles. His mini mental test score is 5. The biochemical results suggest that he has uraemic encephalopathy. How will you manage him?*

A9.2

The principles of treatment are to optimise his diabetic control and treat hyperkalaemia. He should be dialysed for life-threatening states such as hyperkalaemia (after i.v. sodium bicarbonate prior to dialysis), acidosis, fluid overload, pericarditis and encephalopathy. Dialysis may increase, or decrease, body fluids.

Do not dialyse for infection, bleeding, hypermagnesaemia, hyperuricaemia, hypocalcaemia or anaemia. Treat infection with antibiotics and the hypocalcaemia with active vitamin D. The anaemia may be corrected by erythropoietin. The bleeding tendency in ARF may be corrected by a platelet transfusion. The increased neuromuscular excitability is due to hypocalcaemia (which will be exacerbated by bicarbonate infusion) but the possibility of hypomagnesaemia should be considered.

Q9.3 What is the relationship between low magnesium and hypocalcaemia?

A9.3

Magnesium is essential for PTH release and hypomagnesaemia results in resistance to the target organ effects of PTH. The clinical features of hypocalcaemia are the Chovstek's and Trousseau signs. Hypomagnesaemia occurs in 50% of patients on cisplatinum therapy. If the large muscles are twitching, one should consider a dystonia. A past history of phenothiazine use should be elicited.

Q9.4 What is aluminium toxicity?

A9.4

This is dementia caused by aluminium hydroxide binders and should be treated with desferrioxamine. This condition usually affects end stage renal failure patients for several reasons. The kidneys do not lose aluminium as efficiently, dialysate is another source of aluminium and aluminium hydroxide is often used as a phosphate binder.

The diagnosis is made on serum aluminium measurement. Bone biopsy is the gold standard for diagnosis.

The clinical features include, personality change, dyspraxia, speech disturbance, myoclonus and dementia.

The aluminium may accumulate in the bones, causing bone pains, demineralisation and fractures. Treatment is to stop the aluminium and use non-aluminium phosphate binders.

Case 10

Q10.1 What is the most likely diagnosis?

A10.1

Sarcoidosis is most likely because of the skin changes. Usually the lower margin of the hilar nodes is well separated from the hilum in sarcoidosis.

Q10.2 How would you establish the diagnosis?

A10.2

The SACE may be elevated, a positive Kveim test is diagnostic (but waiting for this may delay therapy). Tuberculin is strongly positive at this stage of TB (and, if suggestive, an empirical course of anti-TB therapy should be initiated) but negative in sarcoidosis. Fibre-optic bronchoscopy and transbronchial biopsy may show non-caseating granulomas of sarcoidosis but lymphoma needs exclusion. Mediastin-oscopy and a lymph node biopsy may be the final court of appeal. An associated history of joint pains and goats milk intake requires the exclusion of brucellosis.

Supplementary Question Q10.3   What is the Heerfordt's syndrome?

Supplementary Answer A10.3

This is the combination of fever, parotid enlargement, uveitis and VII nerve palsy in association with sarcoidosis.

Supplementary Question Q10.4   How do you stage sarcoidosis?

Supplementary Answer A10.4

    0 – Normal
    I   – Hilar node involvement
    II – Hilar nodes and parenchyma
    III– Parenchymal infiltration with possible fibrosis

Case 11

Q11.1   What is the diagnosis?

A11.1

This woman has SLE with the anticardiolipin syndrome (antiphospho-lipid syndrome) and had an episode of paradoxical thrombosis on heparin infusion. The VDRL is falsely positive. The lupus anticoagulant test is the *in vitro* prolongation of phospholipid dependent clotting studies. It does not correct with the addition of normal plasma. The antiphospholipid antibodies may also be demonstrated by an anticardio-lipin ELISA. It is possible that immunosuppressive therapy for SLE may predispose to CMV retinitis, which responds readily to gancyclovir but it is more likely that she has cytoid bodies in the perimacular zone.

Q11.2   How would you advise the obstetrician in future pregnancies?

A11.2

Anticoagulation with subcutaneous heparin, low dose heparin and steroids are being used on a trial basis. Due to teratogenicity, warfarin should be avoided during the first trimester.

Q11.3   What is the neurological basis of her symptoms?

A11.3

A large number (10–15%) of SLE patients have cerebral symptoms, which may present as mild neuropsychiatric alterations or forgetfulness. Steroids may rarely cause psychosis but they definitely alter the psyche in subtle ways. Her weakness points to involvement of the contralateral corticospinal tract.

Initially, all these cerebral events were considered to be manifestations of cerebral lupus or a thrombotic event, but studies in Hong Kong suggest that many such patients may have undiagnosed TB of the brain, which may be spotted early by MRI. She may be predisposed to TB of the brain due to her immunosuppressive therapy. In this case ulnar neuropathy should be ruled out as it may be part of the mononeuritis multiplex associated with SLE.

Supplementary Question Q11.4   *How would you detect the presence of the lupus anticoagulant?*

Supplementary Answer A11.4

This is an anticardiolipin antibody which acts as an *in vivo* coagulant but as a test tube anticoagulant. The lupus anticoagulant is also associated with HIV. The presence of an inhibitor will be suggested by a failure of the mixing test to correct the clotting abnormality. The presence of the lupus anticoagulant may be demonstrated by the presence of antibody to phospholipids or the older Russel viper venom test.

Case 12

Q12.1   What has happened and how should it be handled?

Answer 12.1

A test dose of atropine is confirmatory of cholinergic poisoning. The serum erythrocyte cholinesterase level will be low, but there is insufficient time for this test to be clinically useful. The atropine should be given until the wheezing stops, the pupils dilate and there is tachycardia. It should be followed by pralidoxime. It must be emphasised that this cholinesterase regenerator (pralidoxime) must be given early. The same scenario may appear in an agricultural environment. The health carer must remove all clothing and protect himself and the team, as the residue is transcutaneously poisonous. This compound was originally designed for use in war.

Q12.2   What other insecticide is rapidly toxic?

Answer 12.2

In certain parts of Asia, paraquat is used as an insecticide. There is an apocryphal tale of a man who took a sip of this from a coke bottle (not realising that it contained a pesticide) after working in a cemetery. He spat it out immediately. This minute amount of paraquat resulted in oral ulcerations, pulmonary fibrosis and agonising death despite all attempts to save him. These cases are most unfortunate in patients committing parasuicide.

DDT is not as toxic but it accumulates and concentrates over time in the ecosystem. It is stored in fat and cases of death from DDT have been associated with rapid weight loss in obese people.

Case 13

Q13.1   What is the diagnosis?

A13.1

The raised MCV confirms that the woman is still drinking, which may be further supported by a raised γ-glutamyl transferase. This is diagnostic of Wernicke's encephalopathy and peripheral neuropathy in a chronic alcoholic. The combination of thiamine deficiency and carbohydrate intake may cause bleeding into the limbic system. The triad of ataxia, confusion and global nystagmus is diagnostic.

Incidentally, the first case described was of a woman who vomited and did not drink alcohol. One must also consider Wernicke's encephalopathy in non-alcoholics.

Q13.2   What investigations would you perform?

A13.2

Estimation of red cell transketolase may allow biochemical confirmation of the diagnosis. This enzyme is dependent on thiamine pyrophosphate (TPP). The assay is performed with and without TPP. An increase in activity of 30% with TPP indicates deficiency. A rapid disappearance of oedema after i.m. thiamine suggests wet beriberi.

Q13.3   How should this be treated?

A13.3

Treatment with i.v. thiamine will correct the biochemical deficiency, although there may be residual structural neurological damage, which is irreversible. The ECG may show conduction defects with cardiomyopathy.

This may explain some of the cases of Asian's sudden death syndrome, which occurs in foreign manual labourers, who may die from a high cardiac output state. Korsakoff's syndrome may be characterised by an attempt of the mind to fill in the memory gaps with false information, resulting in confabulation.

Case 14

Q14.1 What is the diagnosis?

A14.1

The saturations on the right and left sides of the heart appear normal with no leaks to either side, despite the supranormal high pressure on the right side of the heart which is higher than the left side. This suggests VSD and Eisemenger syndrome.

Q14.2 What would your thoughts be if the catheterisation results were not present and a teenager presented with the same clinical picture and bilateral crackles?

A14.2

One should consider fibrosing alveolitis (if the cough is dry) or cystic fibrosis. The latter may be supported by the presence of a pigeon chest, diabetes (with visual deterioration), retarded growth and an abdominal scar (representing meconium ileus equivalent). The crackles are fine in fibrosing alveolitis but are coarse in bronchiectasis.

Q14.3 What are the normal values for cardiac catheterisation data?

A14.3

	Pressures (mmHg)
RA	4–5
RV	18–30/0–5
PA	18–30/6–12
Pulmonary capillary wedge	6–12

Oxygen values

One need not know the exact values, but the difference between 'blue' and 'red blood' in the various chambers should be mentally visualised as this allows rapid analysis of the cardiac flow pathology. Normally the O_2 content on the right side of the heart should not differ by more than 2% from that of the left side.

Case 15

Q15.1   What would be your immediate action?

A15.1

Administer i.v. crystalline penicillin for the treatment of presumed bacterial meningitis, do an LP (lumbar puncture) after a CT scan, as the size of the fourth ventricle may be a guide to the intracranial pressure. CT scans should be performed more liberally and there is no such thing as a guarded LP.

An emergency thick and thin blood film is needed to search for cerebral malaria, as well as a BM stick analysis of the blood glucose level. Often, when the patient deteriorates on initial therapy for malaria, it is not caused by the parasitaemia, but by the quinine-induced hypoglycaemia. It must be remembered that quinine prolongs the QTc interval (usually less than 10 small squares), and predisposes to torsades de pointes, hence ECG monitoring is essential. Interestingly, cases of malaria have been reported in personnel working at or passing through Heathrow Airport.

Q15.2   What are the causes of hypoglycaemia?

A15.2

Fasting hypoglycaemia is due to excessive insulin secretion such as in insulinoma, mesothelioma and retroperitoneal neoplasms. Insulinoma is the commonest cause of fasting hypoglycaemia in the non-diabetic. Insulinomas are characterised by weight gain. It may also be caused by self administration of insulin.

Fasting hypoglycaemia may also be due to other endocrinopathies such as Addison's and hypopituitarism. Other causes may include alcohol, oral antidiabetic agents, β-blockers, salicylates and liver failure. It is also seen in the terminal phase of renal failure, sepsis and malaria.

Q15.3   How do you differentiate factitious from true hypoglycaemia?

A15.3

This is done by the presence of hypoglycaemia with the simultaneous measurement of the C-peptide. The C-peptide level will be low in factitious cases and the patients are usually from a medical background. This test would have solved the Von Bulow case.

Beware of Munchausen's syndrome by proxy.

Supplementary Question Q15.4   What is the cause of renal failure in malaria?

Supplementary Answer A15.4

This may be due to ATN in falciparum malaria. Several mechanisms are involved. These include intravascular haemolysis with haemoglobinuria (and black water fever), hypovolaemia with renal vasoconstriction and occlusion of small vessels. *Plasmodium malariae* and *P. vivax* may cause a nephrotic syndrome.

Case 16

Q16.1 *What is the diagnosis?*

A16.1

This is the Lesch–Nyhan syndrome. The combination of a raised urate level, choreo-athetosis and self mutilation suggests this diagnosis. Lesh–Nyhan syndrome is due to a genetic deficiency of hypoxanthine guanine phosphoribosyltransferase (HGPRT). Purines may be recycled by extra-hepatic tissues utilising two enzymes of a 'salvage' route. These are the HGPRT pathway and the adenine phophoribosyltransferase (APRT) pathway.

Q16.2 *If the patient is on mercaptopurine for leukaemia and one wanted to prevent a massive urate with a xanthine oxidase inhibitor, how would you titrate the dose of mercaptopurine?*

A16.2

It is critical to halve the dose of mercaptopurine as it will reach a supra-maximal dose in the presence of a xanthine oxidase inhibitor and destroy the bone marrow. This is one of the most dangerous drug interactions in haematology.

Case 17

Q17.1 *What further investigations are indicated and what is the diagnosis?*

A17.1

The failure of the low-dose dexamethasone suppression test to reduce the testosterone level suggest the source is autonomous, and no longer responding to the normal chemical messenger. This excludes polycystic ovarian syndrome and congenital adrenal hyperplasia. The most likely diagnosis is an androgen secreting ovarian tumour. Ovarian ultrasound and venous sampling by catheterising various sites may localise the origin of the neoplasm.

Case 18

Q18.1   Why is the platelet count deranged?

A18.1

It is elevated because the previous accident necessitated a splenectomy for splenic rupture, which may have been diagnosed by peritoneal lavage. Some surgeons fragment the spleen and seed it over the omentum to maintain some defence against encapsulated organisms. Chronic bleeding from occult sites must be sought and polycythaemia rubra vera needs to be excluded.

Q18.2   What are the other causes of such a high elevation of platelets?

A18.2

Myelosclerosis and haemorrhagic thrombocythaemia, in which case the platelets are dysmorphic and dysfunctional. The spleen may be atrophic or absent in sickle cell disease.

Case 19

Q19.1   What is the diagnosis?

A19.1

This is classical of the Fitz–Hugh–Curtis syndrome (which is gonococcal or chlamydial perihepatitis). Adnexal tenderness is present on pelvic examination. There may be pain over the right shoulder. Other associated complications are endocarditis and PUO. One should perform a cervical swab for microscopy and culture, and perform chlamydial serology and blood culture. Urine culture and microscopy should also be performed. The male partner should also be tested and treated, as the pustules and arthritis are highly suggestive of gonorrhoea.

Q19.2   How would you treat this patient?

A19.2

She should be admitted and given a course of doxycycline and ceftriaxone. If the clinical state does not improve over the next few days on this regimen, one should add metronidazole. Contact tracing is part of treatment but the identity of this patient should not be divulged. Her partners should be informed only that they have been exposed.

Case 20

Q20.1   What is your diagnosis?

A20.1

This woman has cryptococcosis and acquired cystic disease. In cryptococcosis, the lower the WCC the worse the prognosis. The antigen test
for cryptococcus is the most sensitive serological test for detecting
fungus; the India ink test misses 30% of cases. She should be treated
with amphotericin and hydration for two weeks, followed by lifelong
fluconazole. A CT scan is vital, as cerebral lymphoma is common in HIV
positive patients. Toxoplasmosis is unlikely as she is already on
adequate prophylaxis.

Cystic degeneration of the kidneys occurs in most patients with
ESRD. The time course is unpredictable. This is common in haemo-
dialysed patients, as well as in conservatively managed cases and with
peritoneal dialysis. The aetiology is unknown. The cyst may rupture into
the collecting ducts causing haematuria, or into the retroperitoneum
where pain is a presenting feature. Erythropoietin production, paradoxically, is enhanced, explaining the rise in Hb concentration.

Q20.2   What is the importance of diagnosing the cysts early?

A20.2

There is a high incidence of neoplasia within these cysts and some may
be malignant.

Q20.3   What further investigations should be performed?

A20.3

A vigilant monitoring of renal function is vital in view of the toxicity of
the amphotericin in this context. Urine should be sent for culture and
cytology. Imaging of cystic kidneys is difficult if small tumours are to be
identified. Ultrasound, CT scanning and arteriography should be considered. Cystoscopy helps to identify which kidney is bleeding. It must
be remembered that patients with analgesic nephropathy have an
increased incidence of urothelial tumours.

Case 21

Q21.1   What diagnosis is indicated by the test of lung function?

A21.1

The reduction in FEV$_1$/FVC ratio (usually > 70) suggests airflow limitation. The methacoline provocation test indicates airway hyper-responsiveness, suggesting asthma.

It must be emphasised that airway hyperreactivity is not synonymous with asthma.

Q21.2   What may have caused this disorder?

A21.2

Soldering surveillance equipment can result in occupational asthma, which can be caused by fumes emitted from colophony resin in the solder wire, or by isocyanates liberated from the polyurethane coating on the wire.

Case 22

Q22.1   What is the diagnosis?

A22.1

The combination of osteoporosis, elevated ESR, raised serum calcium, elevated phosphate and mild renal impairment point to multiple myelomatosis. This can be confirmed by marrow microscopy, which should demonstrate more than 20% infiltration by myeloma cells. Analysis of the urine will demonstrate Bence-Jones protein and electrophoresis will demonstrate an IgG spike with immunoparesis. Although the stiffness and the raised ESR suggest polymyalgia rheumatica, the biochemical findings do not support this diagnosis. The normal alkaline phosphatase suggest bone resorption with no periosteal reaction and some of the zones of osteoporosis on the skull are fragile to pressure trauma. This is characteristic of multiple myeloma.

The renal impairment in myeloma may be due to amyloidosis, hypercalcaemia or blockage of the renal tubules by the light chains. There is a humoral deficiency due to the immunoparesis, which will predispose these patients to recurrent pneumonia, which may be prevented by pneumovax.

Q22.2   How would you treat this disorder?

A22.2

One may irradiate the lytic lesions. Mithramycin and melphalan may control the neoplasm. The hypercalcaemia should be treated by adequate hydration, followed by diuresis, steroids and pamidronate.

Supplementary Question Q22.3   *What is monoclonal gammopathy of unknown significance?*

Supplementary Answer A22.3

This is not myeloma and less than 5% progress to myeloma. There are no bone lesions and there is no immunoparesis. There will be less than 10% infiltration of the marrow, calcium and phosphate are usually normal, but it is not totally benign. There may be development of amyloidosis, neuropathy and renal tubulopathy due to the precipitation of the immunoglobulin chains.

Supplementary Question Q22.4   What is Waldenström's macroglobulinaemia?

Supplementary Answer A22.4

This is a monoclonal gammopathy involving IgM. The malignant cells are monoclonal B cells. This is a pentamer, associated with a hyper-viscosity syndrome. It is an extremely 'sticky' immunoglobulin. A bleeding tendency may result from the macroglobulin interfering with the coagulation factors and platelet function. The treatment includes plasmapharesis and alkylating agents such as chlorambucil or cyclophosphamide. No treatment is needed for patients without symptoms, or with significant hepatosplenomegaly, lymphadenopathy or anaemia.

Case 23

Q23.1   What is the diagnosis?

Answer 23.1

The ocular neurological features suggest botulism. This is due to a presynaptic block in the neuromuscular junction. It is common with canned foods and honey (in children). Neonatal botulism is common in India, as honey is applied to the umbilicus by some communities. The condition may progress to cardiorespiratory failure and bulbar palsy. One should move him immediately into an ITU, intubate and give antibotulinum toxin i.m. early, even to those who are currently asymptomatic. Abdominal symptoms may be absent.

Possible causes are staphylococcal food poisoning, viral gastroenteritis, the Miller–Fisher variant of Guillain–Barré syndrome but the onset of symptoms is too early. Another remote possibility is tetradotoxin poisoning associated with the Japanese puffer fish. This is a sodium channel blocker and death may occur even with expert preparation of the dish. Highly diluted botolinium preparations are used to control refractory dystonias by neurologists.

Q23.2   Does a past history of recovery from tetanus confer lifelong immunity?

Answer 23.2

No. This is why tetanus toxoid should always be given. The incubation period is about a week. Advanced cases require intubation, neuromuscular paralysis and mechanical ventilation. Remember that drug induced dystonias may mimic tetanus. Dystonia should be treated with procyclidine.

Q23.3   Is there another toxin one should consider in the region?

Answer 23.3

Amanita phylloides is a mushroom which causes fulminant hepatitis in 6–12 hours. The amanitin binds and inhibits RNA polymerase. The time course and clinical picture do not support this diagnosis. This is the reason why there are many bold mushroom pickers, but no old bold mushroom pickers. There is a myth that prolonged cooking of this mushroom will detoxify it. All this will achieve is to ensure that your last meal on this planet is 'soggy'. Mushroom poisoning is not uncommon. There are many young 'amateur botanists' who attempt to cultivate certain kinds of mushrooms for their hallucinogenic properties, as they are not illegal.

It is interesting that many natural plants contain compounds which are structurally related to LSD, and are potentially hallucinogenic. In some cultures, psilocibin is used by the Shaman for religious ceremonies. It has been speculated that the burning of the 'witches' in Salem in the USA may have been due to the contamination of their bread by certain hallucinogenic fungi. This may have produced visions and 'mass hysteria'.

Case 24

Q24.1   What is the diagnosis?

A24.1

This patient has an erythropoietin secreting hepatoma (secondary to hepatitis B or alcoholic cirrhosis), and non-megaloblastic macrocytosis and amaurosis fugax.

The alternative is a hepatoma with pulmonary A-V shunting elevating the RBCs.

One should obtain the γ-glutamyl transferase level to assess his alcohol intake and a red cell transketolase level to exclude beriberi. Vitamin B_{12} and folate levels should also be taken. A CT-guided biopsy to obtain the tissue diagnosis will confirm the microscopic architecture of the neoplasm (as well as an ultrasound examination to view its extent). A combination of TIPPS and propranolol will reduce the portal hypertension. The prognosis for a hepatoma is lamentable, and hepatitis B is a major problem in Hong Kong because of vertical transmission. It is also both sexually and haematologically transmitted with minimal exposure. This was dramatically demonstrated by the long-distance runners who contracted it from a participant with minor scratches, after sharing a common shower during the Mexico Olympics.

Supplementary Question Q24.2   *What are the factors which determine whether a hepatitis B infected patient improves or deteriorates and the possible outcome?*

Supplementary Answer A24.2

These are not known; 10% proceed to one of three possible conditions. These may be a chronic carrier state with no histological changes, chronic persistent hepatitis and chronic active hepatitis. During the first five years of chronic infection, viral replication is high. These patients are HBsAg and HBe Ag positive, but HBe antibody negative, HBs antibody negative and HBc antibody negative. They are dangerously infective.

HBV DNA status is the most sensitive index of viral replication and may be assessed by PCR or Southern blot techniques. Subsequently they may improve by mounting antibody responses to HbcAg (which is not serologically detectable), HBeAg and finally HBsAg. The rise in antibodies correlates with a fall in the antigen titres.

Supplementary Question Q24.3   When do you treat hepatitis B positive patients?

Supplementary Answer A24.3

HBeAg positive patients, chronic active hepatitis: interferon will inhibit viral replication and reduce hepatic inflammation.

Case 25

Q25.1   What is wrong with her and what is the treatment?

A25.1

This woman has a combination of mitral stenosis and pulmonary hypertension. The rise in pressure in mitral stenosis is due to the backlog pressure effect of blood in the pulmonary tree and the proliferation of pericytes. The degree of this 'hardening of the pulmonary vessels' (caused by pericyte hyperplasia) is the main criterion which determines the degree of reversibility of the right sided pressure post-valvuloplasty with an Inoue balloon. The best results are obtained in mitral stenosis in young Asians in whom the rate of progression of rheumatic carditis to mitral stenosis occurs at a younger age. Hence they are a cohort who are physiologically better suited for mitral valvuloplasty. The area of the orifice of the mitral valve may be calculated by the pressure half-time equation or by direct planometry.

One should always perform a transoesophageal echocardiogram (TOE) to rule out the presence of clots in the left atrial appendage prior to valvuloplasty. It is not uncommon to see 'smoke' which is the collection of clumped RBCs, and which is a clinical sign of a tendency to clot.

The mainstay of the treatment of mitral stenosis is still control of the heart rate, to increase the time for blood to enter the left ventricle before the next systolic phase. β-Blockers (or digoxin if the patient is in atrial fibrillation) may be beneficial. Pulmonary congestion in mitral stenosis not due to left ventricular failure. The ECG usually demonstrates fast atrial fibrillation. Hyperthyroidism must be ruled out.

Q25.2   When does one cardiovert electrically for atrial fibrillation?

A25.2

Acute pulmonary congestion in association with sudden onset fast atrial fibrillation requires prompt cardioversion. One may infuse amiodarone via the jugular route during the emergency treatment of left ventricular failure. Amiodarone may cardiovert the atrial fibrillation chemically. Prior treatment with amiodarone will increase the probability of electrical cardioversion. Cardioversion is more likely to succeed if the left atrium is less than 55 mm in diameter and the atrial fibrillation is not longstanding. It is important that the patient is adequately anticoagulated for three months prior to cardioversion and the serum potassium must be normal. Digoxin therapy is not a contraindication for electrical cardioversion.

If the atrial fibrillation is recent, some cardiologists would cardiovert patients after a TOE has excluded a left atrial thrombus.

Q25.3   What if the patient in atrial fibrillation complains of severe abdominal pain with no guarding?

A25.3

One needs to consider mesenteric ischaemia with no peritonitis. An emergency angiography to plan for embolectomy must be performed.

Q25.4   How do you calculate pulmonary vascular resistance?

A25.4

This is the mean pressure between the pulmonary artery and the left atrium divided by the cardiac output. The PVR is normally less than one and a value of more than eight increases the risks from surgery.

Case 26

Q26.1 Why is he breathless?

A26.1

He has bilateral diaphragmatic weakness readily ascertainable by fluoroscopy. This is readily diagnosed clinically by the Litton sign (where the movements of the diaphragm are seen by the shadow cast as it tugs on its points of insertion, when moving normally). Other investigations to be performed are the measurement of transdiaphragmatic pressure, transfer factor, and inspiratory and expiratory pressures.

Supplementary Question Q26.2   What are the possible differential diagnoses of bilateral diaphragm paralysis?

Supplementary Answer A26.2

These are muscular dystrophy, polio, Pompe's glycogen storage disease.

Case 27

Q27.1 What is the likely diagnosis?

A27.1

The rise in aspartate aminotransferase levels is suggestive of ischaemic hepatitis due to anoxic damage occurring at the time of cardiac arrest. He should undergo a Holter follow-up and a 12-lead ECG as well as a stress test.

Case 28

Q28.1 What is the diagnosis and why is the sodium so low?

A28.1

This woman has hypothyroidism and pseudohyponatraemia as they are predisposed to hypercholesterolaemia and SIADH. Hypercarotinaemia and macrocytosis are other features associated with this condition. In myxoedema one sees type II fast fibre atrophy, which is one of the reversible causes of madness (dementia). Incidentally the most common cause of carotinaemia in the tropics is an excessive consumption of papaya.

Q28.2 How will you screen for this disorder?

A28.2

A raised TSH with clinical features of hypothyroidism. Rarely, thyrotoxicosis may be pituitary driven, in which case the TSH may be normal or high. In such patients, the clinical features of hyperthyroidism will predominate.

Q28.3 What is 'apathetic thyrotoxicosis'?

A28.3

In some elderly patients, thyrotoxicosis may present with features suggestive of hypothyroidism. There are very few clinical signs and a high index of suspicion is necessary.

Case 29

Q29.1 What are the possible causes of her heart failure?

A29.1

This is the picture of transfusion haemosiderosis with iron deposition in the myocardium (congestive cardiomyopathy) and anaemia. Iron deposition begins in the heart at the age of five and may cause pericarditis or conduction disorders and cardiac arrhythmias. Paradoxically, there is also enhanced iron absorption from the gut with overloading of transferrin. The major cause of death is due to the heart's inability to cope with the deposition of iron. Chelating agents may remove some iron.

The menstrual cycle may be a form of physiological phlebotomy.

Q29.2 What is the haematological diagnostic profile of thalassaemia minor?

A29.2

There is a disproportionate reduction in MCV relative to the haemoglobin. The other features are target cells, basophilic stippling, reticulocytosis, and elevation of HbA2 and HbF.

Case 30

Q30.1   What do you deduce from these results?

A30.1

This excludes Epstein–Barr virus infection. The interpretation of the heterophile test is based on the premise that heterophile antibodies are removed by ox but not guinea pig kidney cells. Heterophile antibodies present in normal sera are absorbed by guinea pig kidney cells, but not ox RBCs. Heterophile antibodies in patients with serum sickness are absorbed by both antigens.

Q30.2   What is a possible diagnosis?

A30.2

Toxoplasmosis or CMV infection. Toxoplasmosis may be diagnosed by a fourfold rise of the specific IgM, which implies acute infection. This is unreliable if the patient is HIV positive. Infection from the residue of cats' faeces causes a lifelong infection which immunosuppression may reactivate. The course is often self limiting but in HIV or other immuno-suppressed patients one may use pyrimethamine and sulphadiazine. In England, half the population is infected by age 70 years but it is more common in the tropics. Transplacental infection may cause abortion; alternatively, it may produce seizures, chorioretinitis, hydrocephalus, microcephaly and cerebral calcification in the new-born.

Case 31

Q31.1   For what is he being treated?

A31.1

He has hyperchloraemic (normal chloride range 95–105 mmol/l) meta-bolic acidosis because of acetazolamide therapy for glaucoma. The anion gap is normal, excluding another source of anions to account for the acidosis such as lactic acid, ketoacids, uraemia, ethylene glycol, hepatic failure and methanol.

Q31.2   What are the other causes of this biochemical profile?

A31.2

The causes of normal anion gap acidosis may be classified into causes due to gut bicarbonate loss, renal bicarbonate loss, impaired renal hydrogen ion excretion and increased HCl production. The causes associated with gut bicarbonate loss includes diarrhoea, ileostomy and ureterosigmoidostomy.

Increased renal bicarbonate loss may be associated with acetazolamide, proximal RTA, hyperparathyroidism, heavy metals and paraproteins.

Reduced renal hydrogen ion excretion may be due to distal (type I) RTA and type 4 RTA (aldosterone deficiency.)

Increased HCl production may be due to ammonium chloride ingestion or increased catabolism of lysine and arginine.

Case 32

Q32.1   What is the cause of her breathlessness?

A32.1

Fibrosing alveolitis is associated with rheumatoid arthritis, accounting for the shrunken restrictive lung picture. The crackles in pulmonary fibrosis are fine. A history of copious mucopurulent sputum production would support bronchiectasis, which can also give the picture of clubbing and coarse crackles. However, this is not supported by the lung function tests.

Q32.2   How would you confirm this diagnosis?

A32.2

Transbronchial biopsy guided by a fibrescope (but this is often not necessary) would confirm this diagnosis but a CT scan may show the peripheral dense lung picture suggesting fibrosing alveolitis.

Q32.3   What are the causes of reduced gas transfer (TLCO)?

A32.3

These are anaemia (for which a correction factor may be applied), reduced alveolar capillary membrane (such as emphysema), obliterative pulmonary vascular diseases and interstitial lung diseases (such as in the case described above). The KCO is also low in all the described conditions, except in those with low accessible lung volume.

Q32.4   What are the causes of increased gas transfer?

A32.4

These are polycythaemia, left to right intra-cardiac shunts, asthma and as an artefact when there is pulmonary haemorrhage.

Case 33

Q33.1   How would you manage him assuming that he needs an operation?

A33.1

This man has steroid-induced osteoporosis. One should increase his steroid dose to compensate him for the stress of the operative phase and reduce it again postoperatively. One should then begin azathioprine, which is a steroid sparer, yet an excellent immunosuppressant.

Q33.2   What is the significance of the lung function test?

A33.2

Restrictive lung defect, which may be seen in this collagen disorder.

Supplementary Question Q33.3   How do you classify lupus nephritis?

Supplementary Answer A33.3

An aggressive nephropathy may be missed because of a borderline urinary sediment.

The lupus nephritis may present as hypertension, which is difficult to treat.

Class I   normal
Class IIa EM or immunofluorescent evidence of mesangial disease
Class IIb Mesangial hypercellularity
Class III FSGN
Class IV   Diffuse glomerulonephritis (more than 50% of glomeruli involved)
Class V   Membranous glomerulonephritis

Case 34

Q34.1 What is the diagnosis?

Answer 34.1

The TSH is not suppressed despite elevated T_3 and T_4 and the THUT shows a supranormal uptake by the gland, suggesting a phenothiazine-induced elevation of the TBG, which may be confused with thyrotoxicosis. It is also important to remember that chlorpromazine may predispose a person to hypothermia.

Q34.2   What other conditions may produce this biochemical profile?

Answer 34.2

Hereditary TBG excess, clofibrate therapy, pregnancy and contraceptive pills.

Supplementary Question 34.3   How would you recognise the sick euthyroid syndrome?

Supplemetary Answer 34.3

Both the T_3 and T_4 will be low. The TSH will be normal and the reverse T_3 will be higher than normal. There is inadequate conversion of T_4 to T_3.

Case 35

Q35.1   What is the diagnosis?

A35.1

This woman is suffering from delirium tremens caused by alcohol withdrawal imposed by hospitalisation. An arterial blood gas must be taken to exclude hypoxia. Some orthopaedic surgeons prefer the pre- and post-operative phase to involve a lower dose of heparin. This would allow a relatively less bloody operative field but predispose to embolism. Fat embolism must be borne in mind and the blood glucose level should be assessed.

Q35.2   What is the treatment?

A35.2

Delirium tremens may occur 1–5 days after ethanol (or barbiturate) withdrawal.

She should be given 9–12 capsules chlormethiazole (each capsule contains 192 mg) for 24 hours, which is then reduced over five days. Alternatively prescribe diazepam 4–100 mg for two days, then reduce it gradually. There is cross tolerance between these two drugs and alcohol. Any dehydration and electrolyte imbalance should be corrected. Vitamin

B_{12} should be given parenterally and any systemic infection sought and treated.

Q35.3 What questions would you ask her?

A35.3

These are psychologically designed questions to detect problem drinkers. Any two positive responses to these questions strongly suggest an alcohol problem.

Q1 Have you ever felt that you ought to cut down on your drinking?
Q2 Have people annoyed you by criticising your drinking?
Q3 Have you ever felt bad or guilty about your drinking?
Q4 Have you ever needed a first drink in the morning to get rid of a hangover ('eye-opener')?

It is noteworthy that drinking 27 units of alcohol per week for men and 20 units for women carries no long-term health risk.

Case 36

Q36.1 What is the diagnosis?

A36.1

Sub-aortic stenosis. The diagnosis is not hypertrophic destructive cardiomyopathy (HOCM) (where the systolic murmur will be softer on squatting) as there is no jerky upstroke. There is an absence of the systolic anterior motion of the mitral valve. Doppler echo cardiography will reveal a gradient and localise it at the anterior four-chamber view. The treatment depends on the degree of obstruction and the type of sub-aortic stenosis diagnosed. These are: membranous, fibromuscular and tunnel stenosis may require a myomectomy.

It is unlikely in this case but collapses following a meal should alert one to the possibility of the lag storage curve, where the delay in the reactive release of insulin to a glucose load is followed by hypoglycaemia. This may be normal, or represent the early stage of incipient diabetes, liver pathology, thyrotoxicosis or previous gastrectomy.

It is also important to perform a Holter to exclude occult paroxysmal dysrhythmia.

Q36.2 What would you consider if she presented with rectal bleeding and aortic stenosis?

A36.2

Angiodysplasia must be considered but the most common cause of a GI bleed is diverticulosis. The urea level will rise in this condition.

Q36.3   What if this patient has supravalvular aortic stenosis, a highly developed sense of musical ability, hypercalcaemia and a relatively borderline IQ?

A36.3

One should consider Williams syndrome.

Case 37

Q37.1   What did the myelogram show?

A37.1

The CSF findings suggest spinal block. The myelogram shows complete extradural obstruction to contrast flow due to thoracic neurofibromas. He has axillary pigmentation called Crowe's sign, as well as other features of neurofibromatosis, such as *cafe au lait* patches, which are not significant if fewer than five are present.

Q37.2   What other pathology may be associated with this condition?

A37.2

Acoustic neuroma, intracerebral glioma, phaeochromocytoma (which may be detected by a MIBG scan), meningioma, spinal neurofibroma (which may cause scoliosis), and there may be an association with the MEN syndromes.

Q37.3   What is the cause of his visual difficulties?

A37.3

An optic nerve glioma, associated with neurofibromatosis, but the possibility of hypertensive retinal degeneration needs to be excluded.

Case 38

Q38.1   What has happened and what is the treatment?

A38.1

This woman has attempted suicide and the psychiatric registrar should be bleeped because salicylate poisoning is being treated. The low CO_2 is due to the direct stimulation of the respiratory centre. Initially, the kidney removes bicarbonate, normalising the pH and producing compensated respiratory alkalosis. This is the initial and diagnostic presentation of salicylic intoxication.

In the absence of treatment, a picture of combined metabolic acidosis and respiratory alkalosis emerges due to the rising level of the salicylate, depressing the respiratory centre (respiratory acidosis). The hypotension and dehydration impairs renal function and there is accumulation of acetoacetate, lactate and pyruvate. Salicylic acid further worsens the state.

Treatment comprises gastric lavage, calling the local poisons unit for advice, and measurement of the salicylate level. The patient should be admitted for observation of signs of toxicity such as vomiting, tremor, ringing in the ears, hyperventilation and confusion. If the salicylate level is less than 4.3 mmol/l, increase the oral fluids. If it is 4.3 mmol/l or above, activated charcoal or alkaline diuresis should be used. An alternative is urinary alkalinisation in the ITU, haemodialysis or charcoal haemoperfusion. Team effort is essential.

Case 39

Q39.1 What was the original diagnosis and what changes occurred after therapy?

A39.1

This woman had accelerated (malignant) hypertension. The normal urine microscopy and normal IVP excludes primary renal disease. High levels of renin are found in accelerated hypertension and reflect renal damage secondary to the hydraulic trauma to the juxtaglomerular apparatus. The term malignant for this condition is now discouraged.

The further increase in renin is because frusemide depletes body sodium and causes renin release. Diazoxide causes renin release due to the circulating volume consequent on the peripheral vascular volume. ACE inhibitors may have been a good choice of treatment for this patient but one of the possibilities to consider with elevated renin is renal artery stenosis, which may cause a catastrophic deterioration in renal function and is worst when the patient is dehydrated. Hence high levels of renin are considered a contraindication to ACE inhibition. One must also remember the first-dose hypotension, which may be delayed in the prodrug formulation, such as enalapril. β-Blockers are obviously contraindicated in view of the asthma.

Q39.2   What is the significance of the hair growth?

A39.2

Hypertrichosis lanuginosa is associated with diazoxide, minoxidil and cyclosporin, and with occult neoplasms of the bronchus, bladder and rectum. Topical minoxidil is now marketed for baldness.

Supplementary Question Q39.3   The random blood sugar suggested that she may have 'borderline diabetes' mellitus. What should be done now?

Supplementary Answer A39.3

Diazoxide is used to reduce insulin secretion in insulinomas. As a consequence of this property, diazoxide may cause HONK in elderly diabetics and produce an artefactual glucose intolerance. The random glucose should be performed once she is no longer on diazoxide.

Diazoxide dilates only arterial smooth muscle. It appears to act by activation of the potassium channels, leading to hyperpolarisation and relaxation of smooth muscle. The cardiac output may increase and renin secretion is enhanced. The side effects also include salt and water retention.

Supplementary Question Q39.4   How would you treat a hypertensive crisis?

Supplementary Answer A39.4

The drugs recommended are i.v. nitroprusside, which is both a venous and an arteriolar dilator, and i.v. labetalol (which is contraindicated as she is asthmatic) which has both central α-blocking and β-blocking properties. Labetalol is safe in pregnancy and may be started intravenously and converted later to an oral form. A nitrate infusion may lower the BP but is only indicated if there is pain accompanying the hypertensive episode.

Case 40

Q40.1   What was the reason for the failure of the Hb to rise?

A40.1

Vitamin B_{12} is absorbed from the terminal ileum. Such a failure of absorption causes pernicious anaemia and the associated presence of iron deficiency anaemia is possible. A megaloblastic anaemia is not synonymous with B_{12} deficiency as there may be coexistent folate deficiency. A peripheral smear will show hypersegmentation of the polymorphs.

The other features of B_{12} deficiency are non-specific blunting of higher cortical functions, ataxia and peripheral neuropathy. The classic presentation is of sudden collapse while washing one's face due to the lack of visual compensation and decreasing sensation of the lower limbs. There is loss of joint position sense and hyperreflexia.

Q40.2   What are the other causes of macrocytosis?

A40.2

In a bleeding peptic ulcer, the Hb will be low and the MCV is high, as reticulocytes are big cells. A high platelet count and urea level, and a positive faecal occult blood would support this picture. Folate deficiency may also coexist, which may be dietary or due to pregnancy, bowel pathology, phenytoin, methotrexate (for which leucovorin rescue has been designed) or oral contraceptives. The causes of non-megaloblastic macrocytosis include alcohol, myelosuppressive chemicals, and myx-oedema. It must be remembered that folate repletion in the presence of untreated B_{12} deficiency may precipitate subacute combined degeneration of the cord.

Case 41

Q41.1   What is the diagnosis?

A41.1

Strongyloidiasis causing malabsorption.

Q41.2   What investigations would you perform?

A41.2

Multi-stool examination for larval microscopy, strongyloides CFT, duodenal aspirate for the larvae and Beal's string test.

Q41.3   How is this treated?

A41.3

Thiabendazole 25 mg/kg twice daily for three days.

Case 42

Q42.1   What are the likely causes of these stones and their therapy?

A42.1

Chronic infection of urease-producing organisms such as *Proteus* spp. Ammonia produced by the hydrolysis of urea alkalinises the urine and will increase the excretion of acidic compounds, providing the ideal conditions for forming urate stones. Continuous prophylactic antibiotics should be given to suppress infection. It is important to differentiate urate from uric acid stones, as treatment for the latter by alkalinisation of the urine will exacerbate stone formation.

Q42.2   What drugs are relatively safe in pregnancy?

A42.2

The safe drugs are the β-lactamases (such as ampicillin, penicillin and cephalosporins), nitrofurantoin and erythromycin.

Drugs contraindicated in pregnancy includes ciprofloxacillin, fluorinated quinolones, tetracycline, ACE inhibitors and phenytoin.

Case 43

Q43.1   What is the diagnosis and how would you confirm it?

A43.1

This suggests mycoplasma pneumonia, which can produce haemolytic anaemia (with large reticulocytes accounting for the raised MCV) due to cold agglutinins, erythema multiforme and peripheral neuropathy. The rash of mycoplasma may sometimes be non-specific. The diagnosis would be confirmed by demonstration of a positive Coombs' antiglobulin test, cold agglutinins in the sera and complement fixing antibodies to mycoplasma pneumonia in paired sera.

Hyponatraemia would be more suggestive of *Legionella*.

Q43.2   What is the treatment?

A43.2

It is interesting that he began tetracycline (which is the correct therapy for mycoplasma) for presumed plague. The alternative is erythromycin, which may cause nausea and abdominal pain. His symptoms resolved, as did the neuropathy. It is now agreed that the mass hysteria regarding the reported Indian epidemic of plague was a mistake, and many eminent Indian virologists believe that it may have been an atypical manifestation of the hantavirus outbreak, which shares many similarities.

Most patients recover in 10–14 days but the disease may be protracted with cough and persistence of the X-ray appearance for weeks. Relapses may occur. Complications such as lung abscesses and pleural effusions are rare. The failure of the wcc to rise is consistent with this disease.

Q43.3   He celebrated the news that he does not have the plague by drinking some vodka. He began to sweat, retch and collapsed. What has occurred?

A43.3

This is a 'disulfiram'-like reaction associated with metronidazole. Other drugs with this property are cefoperazone, cefamandole and cefotetan. Disulfiram acts by inhibiting the aldehyde dehydrogenase enzyme, which causes the accumulation of toxic acetaldehyde. It is therapy of alcoholism by 'intimidation', and tragic deaths have been associated with this pharmacological interaction. Its side effects occur in the rubber industry, where the phenomenon is well known. The effects may last for several hours and the symptoms may mimic an acute myocardial infarction. Full resuscitative facilities should be available.

Case 44

Q44.1   What underlying problem does this man have?

A44.1

Ankylosing spondylitis and he is likely to be HLA B27 positive (seen in 90% of such patients). The cervical spine tends to be brittle, as it is rigid and fractures easily. The ratio of FEV_1/FVC being over 70% makes it likely that he has fibrosing alveolitis and a look at the CXR may show syndesmophytes (producing the bamboo spine) and bilateral sacro-iliitis.

Q44.2   What bedside tests may be performed to follow up the progression of this disorder?

A44.2

These are: the Schober's test, which should show a separation of the fingers by more than 5 cm; chest expansion, which is normally more than 5 cm; and the distance of the occiput from the wall as the patient stands with his back against it.

Q44.3   How do you analyse back pain?

A44.3

A prolapsed intervertebral disc is an acute event, with pain on bending or sitting, and the straight leg raising test is positive. Between the ages of 20 and 40 years the most common cause of back pain is a simple sprain. However one must consider the possibility of spondylolisthesis. The presentation of spondylolisthesis is insidious and the patient has pain during standing and when extending the limb. This is readily diagnosed by performing a lumbar X-ray examination.

After the age of 50 years, osteoarthritis may present insidiously. There is pain on standing, and the straight leg raising test may be positive. If the osteophytes encroach around the cord, they may cause spinal stenosis. Patients suffering from spinal stenosis may have symptoms of 'spinal claudication'. They can cycle but not walk long distances. An obvious possibility to consider in the investigation is a neoplasm. Spinal stenosis is diagnosed by a contrast CT scan with 3D reconstruction. It is treated by surgical decompression.

Q44.4   What is DISH?

A44.4

This is a condition of exuberant osteophyte proliferation in the elderly, involving particularly the dorsal region. It is often asymptomatic but may be confused with ankylosing spondylosis, as back problems are commoner as one ages. There may be associated soft tissue calcification and spur formation when it is called diffuse idiopathic skeletal hyperostosis (DISH) or Forestier's disease.

Q44.5   How would you manage this disorder?

A44.5

An exercise programme is vital. This does not seem to be a problem with the above patient. The drugs used are NSAIDs for night pains, sulphasalazine and methotrexate. The mechanism of sulphasalazine or methotrexate is not well understood in ankylosing spondylosis. They appear to have nothing to do with their well studied properties.

Methotrexate should be used in an extremely low dose with folate repletion, and regular liver function tests. Sulphasalazine and methotrexate seem to act as immunomodulators, as they reduce the inflammatory markers associated with disease activity. There is speculation that these effects may be used to control other inflammatory joint disorders such as rheumatoid arthritis.

Some patients with ankylosing spondylosis may need orthopaedic surgery and joint replacement. The goal of therapy is to prevent the axial skeleton from being so deformed that the patient needs prismatic lenses to look ahead or is wheelchair bound.

Case 45

Q45.1 What is the likely diagnosis?

Answer 45.1

Water intoxication, since he drank more water than can be filtered by the kidney as a result of what he heard from others that adequate hydration may prevent one of the side effects of ecstasy. This has obviously been going on for a long time. Water intoxication causes the renal loss of sodium and the chronicity of this habit has impaired the renal concentrating capacity of the kidney. This may make difficult the distinction between primary polydipsia and diabetes insipidus. A classical water deprivation test will differentiate between the two states. Hyponatraemia should not be treated with hypertonic saline as this may cause cerebellopontine myelinolysis.

Ecstasy (methoxy-methylene-dioxyamphetamine) is an amphetamine-like designer drug which is hallucinogenic in high dosage, simulating the properties of mescaline or LSD. It has been shown to destroy irreversibly the serotonin receptors in rats. There is no standardisation of dosage or purity and it is more poisonous than mescaline.

Supplementary Question 45.2 How do you differentiate between diabetes insipidus and compulsive water drinking?

Supplementary Answer 45.2

In compulsive water drinking, the plasma osmolarity tends to be less than 290 mosmol/kg as in this case, whereas in diabetes insipidus it is above this figure. If a patient with diabetes insipidus is treated with pitressin, the polyuria and thirst ceases and the urine osmolarity automatically rises. In patients who regularly overload their system with fluids, pitressin has a much milder effect due to their neurotic compulsion to overdrink.

Case 46

Q46.1 What is the diagnosis and may his occupation have any relevance?

A46.1

He has the rare combination of primary biliary cirrhosis, scleroderma,

Raynaud's and fibrosing alveolitis. There is a link between scleroderma and Spanish rape-seed oil. This was publicised several years ago in the popular press. There is also a relationship between scleroderma and aeroplane fuel fumes but this link is tenuous.

Supplementary Question Q46.2   How would you diagnose PBC?

Supplementary Answer A46.2

γ-Glutamyl peptidase, 5′-nucleotidase and alkaline phosphatase iso-enzymes to confirm the hepatic origin of this enzyme. A greatly elevated alkaline phosphatase in the absence of abnormal liver dysfunction suggests Paget's disease of bone, metastatic liver disease or primary biliary cirrhosis (PBC).

Anti-mitochondrial antibodies are seen in 90% of patients with PBC and, when in high titres, they are specific for this disorder. Liver biopsy will demonstrate hepatic granulomas with plasma cells and cholestasis. Some proceed to cirrhosis and variceal bleeding, necessitating a transplant (clinically diagnosed by the 'Mercedes Benz' scar).

Supplementary Question Q46.3   How would you diagnose scleroderma?

Supplementary Answer A46.3

This is a clinical diagnosis. Some of the features include tight facies and pseudoraghades with surrounding telangiectasia due to the thickening of the skin. Radiography of the hand will show subcutaneous calcinosis, a barium swallow will show a flaccid oesophagus, and positive antinuclear antibodies and anti-Scl-70 (anti-topoisomerase I) cas be detected. A complication is aspiration pneumonia owing to the flaccid oesophagus.

Scleroderma may exist in a localised form called morphea. A limited form of scleroderma typified by the acronym CREST (calcinosis, Raynaud's phenomena, (o)esophageal involvement, sclerodactyly and telangiectasia) involves the gut and the lungs in the form of interstitial lung disease or pulmonary hypertension. This is associated with a better prognosis.

Case 47

Q47.1   What are the possible diagnoses?

A47.1

This picture is suggestive of HOCM which is genetically passed down in an autosomal dominant fashion. Ectopics generated during the ventriculogram before the slow pull back, one may show post extrasystolic accentuation of the pressure wave form. The ventriculogram will show the form of a 'ballerina's instep' which is suggestive of the diagnosis. Echocardiographers agree that some of the cases previously diagnosed as HOCM were incorrect as the 'cuts' were taken at an angle, or they may be a variant of humpback ventricle.

It is interesting that there is a predominantly Japanese form of HOCM where the thickening is at the apex. The systolic anterior motion (SAM) is due to the Venturi effect as blood accelerates at the outlet. The Venturi or Bernoulli effect is the drop in pressure as fluid accelerates. This explains the bicycle leaning towards the road after a fast bus has passed by.

Q47.2 What is the relationship of the outflow gradient to the prognosis?

A47.2

Considerable significance has been attributed to the pressure gradient in the past. This is easily demonstrated by cardiac catheterisation. However, the pressure gradient does not always reflect significant obstruction to flow and now appears to have little influence on the symptoms or prognosis in patients with HOCM.

Case 48

Q48.1 What is the diagnosis and what therapy should be instituted?

A48.1

Bacterial meningitis with an encapsulated organism such as pneumococcus (also more common in alcoholics) in the setting of the splenectomy, or meningococcus. He should be started on a dose of 2.4 g/24 h of i.v. penicillin or ceftriaxone.

Q48.2 What is his prognosis?

A48.2

The prognosis in pneumococcal meningitis associated with splenectomy and hereditary spherocytosis is variable. These patients may be left with substantial neurological deficits if treatment is not started early. The clinical features of cerebral oedema and focal neurological deficits (not seen in this case) suggest a poor prognosis.

Case 49

Q49.1   What are the diagnoses?

A49.1

The combination of osteomalacia and nephrocalcinosis is highly sus-
picious of distal renal tubular acidosis (type II). There is no evidence of
malabsorption in this patient and he had an equivocal urine sample in
the presence of only mildly acidic urine with systemic acidosis. These
findings are in keeping with renal tubular acidosis.

Q49.2   How would you confirm your suspicion?

A49.2

The gold standard is to demonstrate failure of urine acidification below a
pH of 5.4 after an acid load. This is usually performed using ammonium
chloride 0.1 g/kg body weight. In renal tubular acidosis there is a failure
to maintain a gradient of hydrogen ions across the distal renal tubule. A
persistent acidic environment results, preventing the calcification of
bone with consequent osteomalacia.

Q49.3   What is Bartter's syndrome?

A49.3

This is a recessively inherited condition, characterised by a failure to
thrive, a normal BP, polyuria and polydipsia. Children present with
mental and growth retardation, nocturnal enuresis and there is a familial
clustering. This is due to a failure to conserve salt and water. The low
potassium, alkalosis, high levels of renin and aldosteronism, as well as a
vasopressin resistant concentrating defect, are features of this condition.
On microscopy, there is hyperplasia of the juxtaglomerular apparatus.

   The aetiology of this condition is unknown but it may be due to
defective tubular sodium handling, angiotensin resistance or excessive
prostaglandin synthesis. These are all postulations and none has been
proven.

   Symptomatic improvements may be achieved by correcting the
electrolyte disturbance by dietary modification, potassium supplementa-
tions or spironolactone. Interestingly, propranolol has been used to
suppress renin, and prostaglandin synthetase inhibitors have been
reported to be useful. Some patients have hypomagnesaemia and may
require supplements.

Case 50

Q50.1   What drug did he receive and what alternatives are there?

A50.1

He received stilboestrol (the oestrogen component causes gynaecomastia and the mineralocorticoid component causes salt and water retention). The alternative is orchidectomy, which is unattractive to most patients. The addition of an antiandrogen such as cyproterone acetate seems to increase the median survival time. The alternatives are leuprolide (which is an antiandrogen that stimulates transiently before it blocks the androgen receptors) or flutamide.

Unfortunately, non-hormonal chemotherapy seems unhelpful. There is a more aggressive approach to the early detection of prostatic cancer in the US compared with British practice. This is a controversial area at this moment. One should remember that the PSA may be elevated after a rectal examination.

Case 51

Q51.1   What is the diagnosis?

A51.1

This is pancytopenia with macrocytosis. The megaloblastic anaemia is due to phenytoin (which may cause folate deficiency), or vitamin B$_{12}$ deficiency. The clinical picture suggests paroxysmal nocturnal haemo-globinuria (PNH) as there was a history of back pain and dark urine. PNH often proceeds to an aplastic process, and reticulocytosis would be a feature of haemolysis (although not present with marrow aplasia).

Another possibility is aplastic anaemia, which may also follow viral hepatitis. It is possible that many cases of aplastic anaemia are postviral. Patients with Down's syndrome have a 20% increase in risk for leukaemia.

Aleukaemic leukaemia is another possibility. The age of peak onset is earlier, and the presentation is usually in the first decade of life. Vitamin B$_{12}$ deficiency may show a megaloblastic process and a marrow aspirate may demonstrate leukaemic blast cells or aplasia.

Supplementary Question Q51.2   What are the other causes of marrow aplasia?

Supplementary Answer A51.2

These are heavy metals such as gold, industrial agents such as benzene, phenytoin, chloramphenicol, and hepatitis C and G.

Supplementary Question Q51.3   How would you treat aplastic anaemia?

Supplementary Answer A51.3

This should be handled by a dedicated specialist unit. Obviously, any identifiable aetiological agent should be stopped, benzene for example, benzene although causality is usually difficult to prove. The various modalities of therapy include stimulation of the marrow with bone marrow colony-stimulating factors, antibiotics to treat infection, cyclo-sporin, antithymocyte globulin, platelet transfusion and bone marrow transplantation.

Case 52

Q52.1   What is the diagnosis?

A52.1

This is toxic shock syndrome. The diagnostic features include pyrexia, rash with desquamation 1–2 weeks after the onset of the illness, shock or postural hypotension, clinical or laboratory evidence of three or more organ system involvement. The liver function tests may be deranged, renal failure may be present and other symptoms may include myalgia and confusion. The blood and CSF culture may be negative. The mechanism appears to be a TSST-1 (enterotoxin F) which increases the sensitivity to endogenous toxins and inhibits liver clearance of endotoxin. TSST-1 is a superantigen which may also contaminate surgical wounds.

Q52.2   What is the management?

A52.2

The immediate priority is to treat the shock by fluid repletion and the use of β-lactamase resistant antibiotics. The acute illness should be treated by the use of the appropriate antibiotics in active consultation with infectious disease and microbiology units. She must never use tampons again and must be reviewed in casualty as soon as possible if there is any suspicion of being ill during the menstrual phase.

Q52.3   What are the criteria for diagnosing this condition?

A52.3

These include a temperature of more than 39°C, widespread erythema-tous macular rash, hypotension with a systolic pressure less than 90 mmHg or a postural diastolic drop, and toxic action on at least three systems. These systems may be affected by diarrhoea, vomiting, elevated

CPK, myalgia or raised urea and creatinine. It may also include thrombocytopenia of less than $100 \times 10^9/l$, drowsiness and confusion. There must also be a local source of infection.

Case 53

Q53.1   What is the diagnosis?

A53.1

This is the adult Fanconi's syndrome, with a picture of generalised tubular defect with proteinuria, generalised aminoaciduria, elevated uric acid clearance and raised phosphate loss, as deduced from the low serum phosphate and impaired acidification of urine. The glycosuria (ants collecting) is of the renal type and a standard glucose tolerance test would have a normal or a flat curve.

Supplementary Question Q53.2   What is the difference between RTA types I and II?

Supplementary Answer A53.2

Renal tubular acidosis (RTA) type I is the distal form (counter-intuitively named). This form is generally associated with the autoimmune diseases such as Sjögren's syndrome and primary biliary cirrhosis. The inability to acidify urine can normally be demonstrated by an ammonium chloride load.

The proximal form, also known as the 'classic form' (RTA type II) may be associated with Fanconi's syndrome and Wilson's disease. In the proximal form, the ammonium chloride loading test is normal.

Type III RTA is described in the older books but does not exist for practical purposes. It is described as a combination of RTA type I and II.

Supplementary Question Q53.3   What is RTA type IV?

Supplementary Answer A53.3

RTA type IV is the commonest form of these disorders, characterised by hyperkalaemic acidosis owing to hyporeninaemic hypoaldosteronism. This may occur with a background of mild CRF with tubulointerstitial disease, reflux nephropathy and diabetes.

The combination of hyponatraemia and hyperkalaemia may mimic Addison's disease but RTA IV is a euvolumic state. An identical state may be produced by NSAIDs, which impair renin and aldosterone secretion. This is in addition to NSAID-induced tubular dysfunction.

One treats RTA IV with fludrocortisone, sodium bicarbonate, diuretics and control of the hyperkalaemia.

Case 54

Q54.1   What is the probable diagnosis?

A54.1

This woman has squamous cell carcinoma (cavitation) with hyper-calcaemia and phrenic nerve palsy causing a raised hemidiaphragm. One must also consider the possibility of reactivated sealed TB producing the haemoptysis caused by the hydrocortisone.

This should be treated with radiotherapy.

Q54.2   How does one treat hypercalcaemia?

A54.2

Squamous cell carcinoma *per se* may cause hypercalcaemia. It should be treated if the calcium level is more than 3.5 mmol/l. Features which suggest a neoplastic aetiology are low plasma albumin, low chloride, hypokalaemia, raised alkaline phosphatase, raised phosphate and a positive radioisotope bone scan.

Therapy involves rehydration with 4–6 litres of normal saline (after assessing the ability of the heart to accept a fluid load), and frusemide 125 mg i.v. over three hours. If there is a neoplastic cause, etidronate or pamidronate may be used. These are crystals which lace the wall of the bone, inhibiting the osteoclasts and preventing leaching of calcium into the bloodstream. In vitamin D intoxication, multiple myeloma or sarcoidosis, hypercalcaemia may be treated successfully with i.v. hydro-cortisone.

Q54.3   What are the other causes of hypercalcaemia?

A54.3

These include malignancy (such as myeloma, squamous cancer of the lung, bony metastases), hyperparathyroidism, immobilisation, milk-alkali syndrome, hyperthyroidism, the use of thiazide diuretics and the rare condition of benign familial hypercalcaemia. Vitamin D intoxication is not uncommon among farmers, who feel that it is good for their cows, and may therefore supplement their own diet.

Case 55

Q55.1   Suggest other diagnoses

A55.1

This man may have diabetes, which would have a fasting blood sugar above 8.5 mmol/l. Polyarteritis nodosa (PAN) is associated with a raised ESR, lung changes and eosinophilia. The hallmark of PAN is the fibrinoid necrosis which is seen as a sliver of pink on one side of a blood vessel. Leukaemia may cause retinal haemorrhage due to the associated thrombocytopenia and anaemia. A bone marrow aspirate is essential.

Q55.2   What are the causes of secondary hypertension?

A55.2

These include Conn's and Cushing's syndromes, coarctation of the aorta, contraceptive pills, congenital adrenal hyperplasia (rarely), phaeo-chromocytoma and renal artery stenosis.

Q55.3   How would you diagnose renal artery stenosis, apart from attempting to listen to a bruit?

A55.3

One may perform a captopril renogram. The goal of the test is to measure the injected renal isotope tracer before and after captopril is given. There will be a decreased isotope uptake on the side of the renal artery stenosis.

Q55.4   What are the dangers of sodium nitroprusside use?

A55.4

Nitroprusside is the drug of choice for accelerated hypertension. It produces NO when in contact with RBCs but must be given by a continuous infusion. In the short term, nitroprusside may cause vasodilatation and hypotension but in the long term (24–48 hours), it may produce cyanide. One may reduce the quantity of cyanide by transforming it to thiocyanate. This is achieved by simultaneous administration of thiosulphate.

Even short infusions may be associated with a rebound hypertension. The symptoms of thiocyanate toxicity are nausea, confusion and frank psychosis.

Case 56

Q56.1   What is the diagnosis?

Answer 56.1

This man has biliary obstruction with Coombs' negative haemolysis due to hereditary spherocytosis. The raised bilirubin produces gallstones. Hyperbilirubinaemia is present because of the blockage of the common bile duct. There is an increased osmotic fragility in hereditary sphero-cytosis, which stabilises with glucose.

Q56.2   What additional history is needed?

Answer 56.2

A family history is vital as it is inherited as an autosomal dominant. However, it may arise from a mutation in the absence of a positive family history. An enlarged spleen should be sought by palpitation. Splenectomy does not cure this state but it reduces red cell destruction.

Case 57

Q57.1   What is the reason for the deranged blood film?

A57.1

This woman has haemolytic anaemia secondary to sulphasalazine therapy. This is more common in those with glucose-6-phosphate dehydrogenase (G6PD) deficiency (which was why treatment for malaria in Tehran resulted in so many cases of jaundice giving the drug a 'bad press'). A Heinz body haemolytic anaemia with red cell fragmentation is occasionally seen with patients on sulphasalazine therapy, even with the normal metabolism of the red cell HMP shunt. Heinz bodies require special preparation to be visible. Haemoglobinaemia and haemo-globinuria are of limited duration since only the older cells are vulner-able. Other agents that may precipitate haemolysis in G6PD deficiency are fava beans and moth balls.

   The blood film in haemolysis shows blister cells. There is an elevated LDH level. Dapsone may cause similar problems (and must be con-sidered in a patient with a similar scenario on therapy for leprosy or dermatitis herpetiformis, which may accompany coeliac disease). Oxidative stresses leading to Heinz body formation occur as a result of lack of NADPH, with methaemoglobin formation, oxidation of the thiol compound glutathione, and oxidation of the sulphydryl groups of haemoglobin with destruction and precipitation.

Case 58

Q58.1   What is the diagnosis and what should be done?

A58.1

Alcohol induced dilated cardiomyopathy. The dilated heart in alcoholics has a better prognosis than when there are viral or idiopathic causes of dilated cardiomyopathy. This patient should have afterload reduction with an ACE inhibitor. He should undergo psychological assessment and be counselled with a view to cardiac transplantation.

If he lapses into cardiogenic shock, an intra-aortic balloon pump (IABP) may be a bridge to buy time for the transplant team. When using this device, one must ensure that an adequate volume of blood is perfusing the leg through which it is catheterised. A contraindication to the use of the IABP is aortic regurgitation.

The IABP is an excellent mechanical treatment for unstable angina. It allows surgical revascularisation to be done later. The IABP functions by augmenting intracoronary blood flow (which is one element of Virchow's triad).

Supplementary Question Q58.2   Can an anti-neoplastic agent cause dilated cardio-myopathy?

Supplementary Answer A58.2

This is common with doxorubicin, which causes dose-related myocardial damage. The risk is particularly high once an accumulated dose of $550 \, mg/m^2$ has been exceeded. Once heart failure occurs, the condition is identical to dilated cardiomyopathy but the progression is more rapid.

Supplementary Question Q58.3   What is the prognosis of dilated cardiomyopathy?

Supplementary Answer A58.3

Once symptoms of heart failure develop, the average five-year survival is less than 50%. The life-span may be prolonged by ACE inhibitors but this is modest.

Case 59

Q59.1   What is she suffering from and how is this confirmed?

A59.1

The patient has Lyme disease. The prodromal symptoms are malaise and musculoskeletal pains. 15% of patients develop frank neurological abnormalities with facial palsies (lower motor neurone VII cranial nerve palsy), cranial polyneuropathy and possibly spinal radiculopathy.

The diagnosis is confirmed by antibodies directed against *Borrelia burgdorferi* which has deer (transmitted by *Ixodes dammini*) as one of its reservoirs. The IgM antibodies rise to a peak after six weeks. Although *I. dammini* is the vector, most people affected by this tick are not infected as most of the vectors do not harbour this spirochaete. Lyme disease is endemic on the western coast of north America.

Ixodes is also the vector for Rocky Mountain spotted fever. RMSF has a characteristic rash and shares many of the clinical features of Lyme disease, but it does not affect the VII cranial nerve. It is ironical that RMSF does not occur in the Rocky Mountains.

Q59.2   What would the CSF show?

A59.2

Lymphocytic meningitis and a low glucose level relative to the blood. Sarcoidosis is a remote possibility, as are all causes of lymphocytic meningitis.

Q59.3   How is this treated?

A59.3

Borrelia burgdorferi is a spirochaete. The organism is sensitive to penicillin, amoxicillin and tetracycline.

If the patient is younger than five years avoid tetracycline. Use amoxicillin or chloramphenicol instead.

Q59.4   What is the Lofgren syndrome?

A59.4

This is acute sarcoid arthritis which is associated with an elevated serum urate. Joint effusions are uncommon in this condition. Sarcoidosis is one of the causes of VII cranial nerve palsy.

Case 60

Q60.1   What is the explanation for the biochemical changes?

A60.1

The calcium level was not adequately depressed following a ten-day course of hydrocortisone (40 mg eight hourly) and is consistent with primary hyperparathyroidism.

About half of tumour-associated hypercalcaemia fails to be suppressed with glucocorticoids and is responsive to etidronate. It cannot be overstressed that hypercalcaemia is a medical emergency and requires prompt therapy. All other forms of hypercalcaemia may be suppressed with steroids. The differential diagnoses in this case are sarcoidosis, hypervitaminosis D, tumour and thyrotoxicosis.

Q60.2   What are the situations requiring corticosteroid treatment in sarcoidosis?

A60.2

Corticosteroids may be used in sarcoidosis if there is cardiac involvement, progressive lung disease, neurological sarcoid or eye involvement. It may also be used in acute extensive lung infiltration with symptoms or hypercalcaemia *per se.*

Q60.3   How would you diagnose sarcoidosis?

A60.3

Erythema nodosum and bilateral hilar lymphadenopathy in a youth may be sufficient to make a diagnosis. The other supportive markers are a raised ESR, hypercalcaemia and hypercalciuria.

The serum level of ACE is raised. The SACE level is raised in 60–80% but this is less helpful in atypical presentations of sarcoidosis. Incidentally, serum ACE is also raised in other granulomatous and chronic inflammatory disorders. Unfortunately, ACE levels are not as useful as was originally hoped in the diagnosis of sarcoidosis.

Biopsy of appropriate tissue with a characteristic granuloma will confirm the diagnosis. This may be combined with a broncho-alveolar lavage, which shows an elevated number of activated T-lymphocytes. The broncho-alveolar lavage picture may be simulated by other conditions such as extrinsic allergic alveolitis.

A gallium scan may detect zones of active sarcoidosis as it is taken up by active macrophages. The gallium scan is not specific but can be useful in assessing the activity of sarcoidosis.

Supplementary Question Q60.4   How would you treat sarcoidosis?

Supplementary Answer A60.4

No specific treatment may be necessary since spontaneous resolution may occur. Mild symptoms may be alleviated by NSAIDs. Steroids are useful as they promote the healing of granulomas and produce short-term resolution, although their effect on the natural history of the disease is uncertain. Once systemic steroids are initiated, they are often necessary for 1–3 years in suppressive doses of 5–15 mg daily. Other drugs which are used are hydroxychloroquine for cutaneous sarcoidosis, and azathioprine and methotrexate in severe disease.

Case 61

Q61.1 What is the diagnosis and the treatment?

A61.1

Klinefelter syndrome presents with gynaecomastia and subnormal development of the genitalia (small testes and penis). The results show a pattern of hypergonadotrophic hypoganadism. The deficiency of androgens allows excessive growth of the long bones and this is responsible for their limbs in relation to total height. There is a female hair distribution. Testicular biopsy shows fibrosis and hyalinisation of the seminiferous tubules and results in small firm testes and azoo-spermia. Chromosomal analysis shows a characteristic karyotype of 47XXY, but some patients are mosaics with a combination of 46XY/47XXY and may be fertile.

Therapy is by testosterone injection given by monthly depot, which increases virilisation and improves symptoms of androgen deficiency; it prevents osteoporosis but will not restore fertility.

Q61.2 What is the incidence of this disorder?

A61.2

This is the most common of the genetic diseases involving the sex chromosomes. The occurrence is one in 600 American live births. It is one of the most common causes of hypogonadism in males.

Case 62

Q62.1 What is the diagnosis?

A62.1

Polycythaemia rubra vera. Pruritis in the absence of such a fever should also alert one to the possibility of an occult lymphoma. Another entity is the Gaisboeck's syndrome (which is not associated with itching), which has an uncertain aetiology. This is usually seen in overweight executives who smoke a great deal and drink an excess of alcohol (the treatment of which is not rehydration but change of lifestyle). One should also rule out any causes of chronic hypoxia (although the elevated WCC makes this unlikely) such as bronchitis or an AV fistula.

Q62.2 How would you confirm the diagnosis?

A62.2

The diagnosis is confirmed by demonstrating a red cell count, an elevated red cell mass and normal arterial blood gases. The marrow is increased with greater red cell mass, and more myeloid cells and megakaryocytes. Neutrophil alkaline phosphatase staining is increased. Marrow stores are depleted of iron. Severe chronic obstructive pulmonary disease is the most common cause of secondary polycythaemia and should be excluded by clinical examination and lung function tests.

Q62.3 What are the therapeutic options?

A62.3

Treatment includes phlebotomy, ^{32}P irradiation (which is associated with a increased risk of leukaemia), cytotoxic drugs, hydroxyurea (which is non-mutagenic) and α-interferon. Anagrelide may be used to control thrombocytosis. Polycythaemia rubra vera may lead to extramedullary haemopoiesis. This may produce a large spleen which in time may lead to myelofibrosis. The clinical picture may be confused with chronic myeloid leukaemia.

The LAP score is elevated in polycythaemia rubra vera but decreased in chronic myeloid leukaemia.

Supplementary Question Q62.4   What is the significance of the pruritis?

Supplementary Answer A62.4

The pruritus is related to raised circulating histamine due to an increase in basophils which degranulate. This is also associated with peptic ulcer disease. The basophil level is usually less than 1×10^9/l but is significantly elevated in myeloproliferative disorders.

Case 63

Q63.1   What is the cause of the visual problem?

A63.1

In multiple sclerosis the CSF will demonstrate an oligoclonal band and the MRI will show zones of demyelination. Progressive multifocal leucoencephalopathy (PML) caused by the JC virus will appear similar in HIV patients. The course of PML is more rapid than multiple sclerosis and there is a median survival of six months once it becomes manifest. The Devic's variant of multiple sclerosis seen in Asians has a better prognosis and is more common nearer the equator.

About 40–60% of patients with optic neuritis develop full blown multiple sclerosis. Acuity returns to normal over a few months but there is usually a residual impairment of colour vision. On fundoscopy, the temporal half of the optic disc which contains the macular fibres may be pale. Patients with HLA-DR2 and those with more than one attack of winter-onset optic neuritis are more likely to progress to full blown multiple sclerosis. Steroids may reduce the plaque oedema but will not alter the progression of the disease. The 'barber chair sign' is usually elicitable in such patients. The weakness of the leg may be due to a plaque in the cord.

Case 64

Q64.1   What is the reason for the biochemical picture seen?

A64.1

The plasma creatinine is high relative to the urea in this patient. This may be due to his low protein diet despite his chronic renal failure. Urea derives from protein, the reduction of which will translate into a fall of the urea/creatinine ratio. His liver enzymes should also be screened because a hepatic inability to metabolise amino acids to urea is another cause and hepatitis A and E are common in the regions he visited.

Q64.2   In what other conditions may this disparity be found?

A64.2

Other causes for a fall in the urea/creatinine ratio are seen in starvation, and in haemodialysis or peritoneodialysis. Both these procedures remove urea more effectively than creatinine because urea has a lower molecular weight and is more easily cleared.

This condition is also observed in hyperemesis gravidarum and pyloric outlet obstruction owing to a neoplasm, where constant vomiting reduces the amount of urea absorbed. Urea is lost more than creatinine in the vomitus due to its capacity to diffuse more pervasively into all parts of the body. In severe liver failure, the figures would be lower, such as a urea of 2 mmol/l and a creatinine of 149 µmol/l.

Case 65

Q65.1   *What are the possible causes of the CXR changes?*

A65.1

One should still consider TB despite the negative AAFB in the sputum. The sputum should be sent for culture. A full TB screen should also consist of three samples of early-morning urine, stained for AAFB. The combination of eosinophilia, upper lobe shadowing and the asthma with chronic sputum production makes allergic bronchopulmonary aspergillosis (ABPA) likely. Some asthmatics develop a sensitivity to the fungus *Aspergillus fumigatus*. This mould lives on rotting vegetation. The CXR may show patchy infiltration and areas of collapse, fibrosis and bronchiectasis. The airway may be blocked by masses of fungal hyphae.

The radiological changes make other causes of bronchopulmonary eosinophilia less likely. A diagnosis of ABPA would be supported by a positive skin test and the presence of precipitins to *A. fumigatus*. The organism may be isolated by fibre-optic bronchoscopy with bronchial lavage and bronchial biopsy. On the other hand, a caseating TB granuloma or, rarely, Churg–Strauss syndrome, may be diagnosed. Churg–Strauss syndrome is a vasculitis which usually spares the kidney.

Q65.2   *What are the features of an acute severe attack of asthma?*

A65.2

- Inability to walk
- Inability of the patient to speak in complete sentences
- Cyanosis
- Lack of wheezing (owing to poor air entry)
- Respiratory rate > 25/min
- Pulse rate > 110/min
- Peak flow rate < 200 l/min or 50% < than normal
- Pulsus paradoxus (> 15 mmHg)

Q65.3   *How would you manage an acute attack of asthma?*

A65.3

Give maximum oxygen with a nebulised β-agonist. The nebulised β-agonist may be given at 15-minute intervals in severe cases. Nebulised ipratropium bromide should be added to the nebuliser if the response to the first β-agonist is not satisfactory. Intravenous hydrocortisone should be given and, if nebulised bronchodilators are not effective, one should give i.v. salbutamol or aminophylline. If the patient is taking aminophylline at home, do not give a loading dose.

Steroids, β-agonists and hyperventilation will all reduce the serum potassium, which should be monitored and replaced. Often, asthmatic patients are dehydrated and will need i.v. fluid replacement. If the blood gases deteriorate, particularly if the $PaCO_2$ is normal and the oxygen is low, this is highly suggestive of an impending respiratory arrest and ventilatory support should be considered. The severity of asthma is usually underestimated.

An acute attack of asthma should be regarded as a failure of routine management. The reasons for failure should be explored.

Case 66

Q66.1   What is the diagnosis?

A66.1

Reiter's syndrome (reactive arthritis following an episode of dysentery). In post-dysenteric dysentery, the arthritis occurs approximately two weeks after the initial symptoms. Weight-bearing joints are particularly affected asymmetrically and may have effusions. One must rule out gonococcal arthritis and if there is doubt, there should be a diagnostic aspiration. The urethritis in Reiter's syndrome is mild and may be detected using the two-glass urine test. Ocular and skin involvement with pustular psoriasis of the soles (keratoderma blenorragica), circinate balanitis and pleurisy are rarer manifestations of the syndrome. Reiter's first case was a cavalry officer.

There is a well-known case of a naval ship where a large number of the crew had infectious diarrhoea. The members of the crew were followed up on recovery and it was found that a large number who subsequently developed sero-negative arthropathy had HLA B27. This was an accidental but informative experiment on an isolated group of young men.

Q66.2   What organisms are implicated?

A66.2

- *Shigella flexneri*
- *Salmonella typhimurium*
- *Yersinia enterocolita* – particularly associated with terminal ileitis as in this case
- *Campylobacter*

Amoebic dysentery has recently been linked to this syndrome.

Q66.3   Is this a sexually transmitted disease?

A66.3

In the UK and the USA most cases follow intercourse, but in Europe dysentery is reported to be the more frequent precipitating event.

Q66.4 How do you analyse a joint aspirate?

A66.4

Never aspirate a joint if the overlying skin is infected. The joint may be normal and the aspiration will introduce infection. Normal joint fluid is straw-coloured and clear to light in a test tube. One used to test its consistency by the ability to stretch it between two fingers (called the 'string sign' due to the presence of hyaluronate). This is no longer done for obvious reasons. One would then send it for culture, examine it for white cells and crystals (e.g. in gout, the crystals are yellow when viewed through a polarising microscope, and by convention are described as having a negative birefringence).

If there are less than 25 000 cells/mm^3 the condition is non-inflammatory, as in osteoarthritis or trauma. In rare cases, if the cells are around 25 000/mm^3 but mainly lymphocytes, one should consider TB and stain the aspirate with Ziehl–Nielsen followed by a culture.

If there are between 25 0000 and 100 000 cells/mm^3, this is an inflammatory exudate, the differential diagnosis of which includes rheumatoid arthritis, SLE, gout, pseudogout and psoriatic arthritis.

If there are more than 100 000 cells/mm^3, this is a septic arthritis and the differential diagnosis includes a staphylococcal or gonococcal arthritis.

Case 67

Q67.1 What is the diagnosis?

Answer 67.1

Acute viral meningitis with coxsackie myocarditis (usually Coxsackie B virus group). Chagas disease is a possibility in view of his South American origin, but this does not cause meningitis.

Q67.2 What other organisms may cause this picture?

Answer 67.2

Echovirus, mumps, EBV (infectious mononucleosis).

Q67.3 What less common disorder may produce a similar picture?

Answer 67.3

Q fever, leptospirosis, leukaemic meningitis, Behçet's and TB meningitis. Other chronic bacterial infections are not likely because the CSF sugar is more than 40% of the blood sugar, which is normal.

Case 68

Q68.1 What is the diagnosis?

A68.1

Dubin–Johnson syndrome which is a chronic benign intermittent jaundice with conjugated hyperbilirubinaemia and bilirubinuria.

Q68.2 How will you confirm it?

A68.2

Bromosulphaphthalein test in which, after an initial fall, there is a secondary rise after 120 minutes, which is higher than the 45 minutes slope. A liver biopsy will show a greenish black liver with melanin. This is a genetic defect in the canalicular transport of organic ions.

Q68.3 What is the prognosis?

A68.3

Excellent, after she stops the oral contraceptive, but she must be warned that it may recur during pregnancy.

Case 69

Q69.1 What is the diagnosis?

A69.1

Pulmonary stenosis and an ASD with a left to right shunt. The pulmonary stenosis is demonstrated by the much lower pressure between the pulmonary artery and the right ventricle. A gradient across the pulmonary valve is not clinically significant unless the pressure difference is more than 20 mmHg.

Q69.2 What would a CXR show?

A69.2

The CXR may show a prominent pulmonary artery due to post-stenotic dilatation.

Case 70 ✓

Q70.1 What is the diagnosis?

A70.1

This is seronegative polyarthritis and the presence of PAS positive matter in the macrophages of the small bowel biopsy makes Whipple's disease likely. 60% of such patients have rheumatological manifestations before their gut symptoms appear. On electron microscopy, bacilli may be seen within the macrophages. The name of the organism is *Tropheryma whippelii*.

Q70.2 How should his arthritis be treated?

A70.2

The arthritis is unresponsive to gold or penicillamine and settles following a long course of penicillin, erythromycin or tetracycline. If the patient fails to improve, one should consider using an antibiotic that crosses the blood–brain barrier, such as chloramphenicol.

Q70.3 How do you classify diarrhoea?

A70.3

One breaks it down to bloody and non-bloody diarrhoea. If there is no blood, consider preformed toxins such as *Bacillus cereus* and *Staphylococcus aureus*, viruses and protozoal infections. The causes of protozoal induced diarrhoea are *Giardia* (common in St Petersburg), cryptosporidiosis (common in HIV patients) and microsporidiosis. The causes of bloody diarrhoea are *Clostridia*, *Campylobacter*, *Salmonella*, *Shigella*, *Yersinia*, *E. coli* and *Vibrio*. Beware of 'holy water' from obscure sources because cases of amoebiasis have been reported in this context.

Supplementary Question Q70.4   What are the other manifestations of Whipple's disease?

Supplementary Answer A70.4

It may present with steatorrhoea, as in this case, along with symptoms of fever and weight loss. Peripheral adenopathy, and involvement of the heart, lungs and brain may occur.

Case 71

Q71.1 What is the diagnosis and how does this condition occur?

A71.1

This woman has anticonvulsant osteomalacia, accounting for the back-ache. Phenytoin tends to cause coarsening of facial features, which is why it is relatively contraindicated in young girls. This form of iatrogenic osteomalacia is seen with phenytoin and phenobarbitone used chronically. Phenytoin causes hepatic enzyme induction.

The mechanism is a non-specific induction of the liver, which impairs vitamin D_3 hydroxylation, producing paradoxically more polar inactive metabolites. There is therefore less 25-OHD$_3$ to be further hydroxylated to 24,25-di-OHD$_3$ and subsequently to 1,24,25-tri-OHD$_3$. The physiological function of 1,24,25-tri-OHD$_3$ is to promote gut absorption of calcium. When there is a lack of active complete vitamin D, the calcium level drops and osteomalacia develops. In chronic biliary cirrhosis, similar vitamin D abnormalities are seen and osteomalacia may occur.

Supplementary Question Q71.2   What the other drugs cause hepatic enzyme induction?

Supplementary Answer A71.2

These include the other anticonvulsants, e.g. antibiotics such as rifampicin, barbiturates, meprobamate, carbamazepine and primidone. Other enzyme inducers include chronic alcoholism, barbecued meat and Brussels sprouts. The miscellaneous causes are tobacco, sulphinpyrazone, DDT, glutethimide and griseofulvin.

Supplementary Question Q71.3   What are the other side effects of phenytoin?

Supplementary Answer A71.3

Phenytoin may also cause neurological symptoms such as confusion, ataxia and acute diplopia. Other associated side effects are the Steven–Johnson syndrome, hirsutism, gum hypertrophy and aplastic anaemia.

Case 72

Q72.1 What are the diagnoses?

A72.1

Diabetes mellitus and acromegaly with bitemporal hemianopia (in which a lateral skull radiograph view will demonstrate the bloating of the sella turcica). This explains his loss of fighting skill. In a normal person, a glucose load lowers the growth hormone to 4mU/l but in acromegaly, it may paradoxically rise.

As per WHO criteria, a fasting venous level of more than 7.8mmol/l of glucose is IGT and a level of 11mmol/l is diabetes mellitus. Half of patients with acromegaly have problems coping with sugar handling (20% have diabetes and another 30% have impaired tolerance).

The changes of acromegaly are so insidious that those close to these patients may not notice anything, but serial comparison of past photographs will unveil the changes.

His numbness is suggestive of carpal tunnel syndrome. This may be clinically diagnosed by Tinel's sign, Phalen's test and a weakness of the abductor pollicis.

Q72.2   What happens to the GFR, the phosphate and the urinary calcium level?

A72.2

They are all elevated.

Q72.3   What are the causes of death in this disorder?

A72.3

These are cardiac failure, hypertension and myocardial infarction.

Supplementary Question Q72.4   How would you treat this patient?

Supplementary Answer A72.4

This patient needs either yttrium implants or a surgical resection. His diabetes and hypertension needs to be controlled. Specific therapy includes somatostatin and bromocriptine. He will also need an assessment of his coronary reserve.

Supplementary Question Q72.5   What is the role of IGF-1?

Supplementary Answer A72.5

It aids the diagnosis of acromegaly as it reflects the mean 24-hour growth hormone level.

Case 73

Q73.1   What possible diagnoses would you consider?

A73.1

TTP, SLE and other collagen diseases should be considered. TTP (Moschcowitz's syndrome) is characterised by microangiopathic haemolytic anaemia and thrombocytopenia, neurological, renal disease and fever. Renal changes are due to the hyaline adjustments with occlusion and proliferation of the glomeruli. The blood film will show schistocytes (fragmented cells). The antiglobulin test is negative with thrombocytopenia and there is a prolonged bleeding time. There is no evidence of DIC and a leucocytosis with a left shift may occur.

Case 74

Q74.1   What is the diagnosis?

A74.1

Leptospirosis. They were all attempting to escape through a concealed tunnel, which was flooded with contaminated sewage. Leptospirosis may progress to renal failure and myocarditis. Transmission is via rat urine as well as dog and livestock urine. By the time the meningeal symptoms appear, the organisms have disappeared from the CSF. There is a non-icteric form associated with myalgia, headache, abdominal pain, vomiting, fever and uveitis.

Q74.2   How would you confirm it?

A74.2

Blood culture in Fletcher's medium and examination of urine for Leptospira. The organism is a spirocheate (*Leptospira interrogans* complex), which may be visualised through a dark field microscope. Doxycycline or tetracycline may be used to cover short-term exposure of the staff who were in contact with the tunnel and the patients. The definitive therapy is penicillin G or tetracycline. Rat control should be initiated and an infectious disease team should be deployed to the island.

Q74.3   What is the prognosis?

A74.3

Overall, the prognosis is good if there is adequate early treatment. Attention to fluid balance and dialysis may be necessary. The poor prognostic indicators include severe jaundice, DIC, renal failure and respiratory failure.

Case 75

Q75.1 Suggest two possible diagnoses and their management.

A75.1

The absence of cardiac enlargement suggests a pulmonary cause for this pathology. Any past pelvic operation would raise the possibility of a pulmonary embolism (PE) but this picture is classical of fibrosing alveolitis. Other forms of fibrosis such as sarcoidosis and lymphangitis may present in the same way. Sputum must be screened for neoplastic cells, and lung function tests carried out to measure FEV_1, FVC, transfer factor and lung compliance.

If multiple PE is suspected, this would be reflected in echocardiography as RV strain. Fragments of the clot may be seen by TOE. A lower-limb venogram, Doppler or a *V/Q* scan may well diagnose a PE. The gold standard is still angiography. Tests for allergens are skin tests, avian precipitins and the Kveim test for sarcoidosis.

In cor pulmonale one should give diuretics, digoxin, and 100% O_2. In extrinsic allergic alveolitis, steroids are indicated together with anticoagulation.

Case 76

Q76.1 What is the diagnosis?

A76.1

This patient has pericarditis characterised by a saddle-shaped ST elevation (instead of the cathedral type of ST elevation seen in an acute infarct). The ST elevation is seen in most leads, rather than the localised pattern seen in ischaemia, as this is a generalised inflammation. The arthralgia is due to drug-induced SLE, which does not affect the kidneys.

Q76.2 What blood tests would you perform?

A76.2

Measure the ENA, and DNA antibodies, which should be negative in a drug-induced SLE. Antihistone bodies are the *sine qua non* of drug-induced lupus.

Supplementary Question Q76.3 What other drugs may produce lupus?

Supplementary Answer A76.3

Hydralazine, isoniazid and procainamide are the most likely causes in slow acetylators. Any phenotype may have an SLE like syndrome may occur in all phenotypes with cardiological drugs such as β-blockers, amrinone, captopril and quinidine. The other causes are chlorpromazine, phenytoin, clonazepam and some sulpha drugs. The syndrome usually disappears when the drug is withdrawn.

Supplementary Question Q76.4   What is the prognosis for SLE?

Supplementary Answer A76.4

The course is episodic with exacerbations and remissions that may last for long periods. This may also occur in patients with renal disease. The early estimates of the mortality were exaggerated but the five-year survival rate is about 95%. In most cases the pattern of the disease becomes established in the first few years after presentation. If serious problems have not developed by this time, they are unlikely to do so.

Case 77

Q77.1   What is the diagnosis?

Answer 77.1

Carcinoid syndrome due to an elevated 5-HIAA (5-hydroxyindoleacetic acid). The normal excretion of 5-HIAA is 2–10 mg/day but this may rise above 50 mg/day in carcinoid syndrome. The right heart failure may be due to pulmonary stenosis. The right hemicolectomy was an attempt to resect the tumour. The florid presentation of this patient suggests that the carcinoid has seeded the liver and beyond.

Case 78

Q78.1   What is the diagnosis?

A78.1

Lag storage response. This is associated with thyrotoxicosis, when the glucose level peaks at 30 min, and then falls below normal levels by 90 minutes. The insulin response is retarded despite the excessive glucose flood, causing glycosuria. This is another reason why the urinary estimation of blood glucose is unreliable.

Q78.2   In what other conditions may this be found?

A78.2

It may also be seen in normal people, before the onset of full blown diabetes, post-gastrectomy, and in liver disease (due to decreased glycogenolysis).

Case 79

Q79.1   What are the possible diagnoses?

A79.1

Ventricular aneurysm, which may be suggested by a persistently raised ST segment in the lateral precordial leads, mitral incompetence due to ruptured chordae tendinae (or infarction of papillary muscle) and a VSD due to ischaemic necrosis of the septum.

Q79.2   What investigations would you perform?

A79.2

CXR, echocardiography and cardiac catheterisation with a ventriculogram.

Q79.3   What is the prognosis?

A79.3

Usually good, as all these conditions are amenable to surgical intervention. In a post-infarct VSD, one may decide to delay the repair until the zone of necrosis is clearly demarcated. This makes it easier to suture with either a Dacron or a pericardial patch over the hole. There is another school of thought that believes in early intervention when the patient is in the best physiological state before damage to other life support organs have occurred.

Q79.4   What does the fever, pleural rub and leucocytosis suggest?

A79.4

These features suggests a large infarct.

Q79.5   The 12-lead ECG demonstrated a RBBB pattern of pacemaker capture. What is your diagnosis?

A79.5

She has developed a VSD, and the pacing wire is pacing the left ventricle.

Case 80

Q80.1 What is the diagnosis?

A80.1

Guillain–Barré syndrome is a typical symmetrical ascending paralysis with a history of viral infection, which clears by the time the neuropathy appears. Sphincter involvement is common and muscle pain is seen in 30% (but less severe than in poliomyelitis, which is usually asymmetrical with the CSF suggesting a lymphocytic meningitis). There may also be features of autonomic dysfunction and the CSF is characterised by an albuminocytologic dissociation in which the protein is elevated but not the cells. The above case exemplifies a rare variant associated with ataxia and initially involves the ocular muscles, known as the Miller–Fisher syndrome.

Supplementary Question Q80.2   What are the principles of treatment of this disorder?

Supplementary Answer A80.2

High-dosage i.v. γ-globulin reduces the duration and severity of the condition. Mechanical ventilation may be necessary. Plasmapheresis has been proved to be beneficial in reducing the period of disability. Complete recovery may gradually occur over many months. Recovery may sometimes be incomplete. Corticosteroids are used in therapy but they are not proved to alter the course of the disease.

Supplementary Question Q80.3   What are the differential diagnoses?

Supplementary Answer A80.3

Spinal cord block (Froin's syndrome) may cause greatly elevated protein levels alone. This may be documented by the alterations in CSF pressure changes during respiration.

A cauda equina lesion may be suggested by flaccid paralysis and there is loss of sphincter tone and back pain. Polymyositis may be excluded by a normal CK estimation. There are no cutaneous changes such as a heliotrope rash, nail fold vasculitic lesions and Gottron's papules over the dorsum of the knuckles, which are associated with dermatomyositis.

Supplementary Question Q80.4   *What investigation is it critical to observe continuously?*

Supplementary Answer A80.4

Spirometry is important because this syndrome is a known cause of neurogenic hypoventilation (the blood gases deteriorate late in Guillain–Barré syndrome).

Supplementary Question Q80.5   *What if this patient has papilloedema with visual blurring?*

Supplementary Answer A80.5

The elevated proteins can occlude the arachnoid villi and cause pseudo-tumour cerebri.

Case 81

Q81.1   *What operation was performed?*

A81.1

He underwent ureterosigmoidostomy, in which hydrogen chloride was absorbed, resulting in hyperchloraemic acidosis. Potassium is not absorbed to any extent and the bowel may excrete excess potassium due to mucosal irritation by the urine. It is also possible that he had a renal stone removed for renal tubular acidosis.

Q81.2   *What is the other explanation for this picture?*

A81.2

In RTA, there is a failure to lose acid, hence the value of the urinary acidification test. There is failure to maintain a normal gradient of hydrogen ions in the distal tubule, hence the reduced bicarbonate excretion and consequent metabolic acidosis. The anion gap left by the reduced bicarbonate is filled by chloride anions. This is therefore a normal anion gap acidosis.

Normally, sodium is exchanged for potassium in the distal tubule. In RTA, there are insufficient hydrogen ions available (as the gradient is not maintained) and potassium is sacrificed in the exchange mechanism, causing hypokalaemia. The hyperkalaemia explains his chronic fatigue.

Case 82

Q82.1   What was the diagnosis?

A82.1

There is an inadequate response to synthetic ACTH (normal being an increment of at least 190 nmol/l with the serum cortisol rising to at least 500 nmol/l). This suggest iatrogenic adrenal insufficiency caused by the high steroid dose taken for his asthma.

Case 83

Q83.1   What is the diagnosis?

A83.1

Paroxysmal nocturnal haemoglobinuria (PNH).

Q83.2   What happens a few weeks later?

A83.2

Budd–Chiari syndrome (hepatic venous obstruction). In time, hepato-megaly and ascites will develop. An inferior venous injection of contrast will show the characteristic distortion of the vein throughout its intra-hepatic course.

Q83.3   What additional investigations are required?

A83.3

Blood and urine should be examined for free haemoglobin.

Q83.4   What confirms the diagnosis?

A83.4

The Ham test. The RBCs in PNH are more easily haemolysed in an acidified medium than normal. The term nocturnal is a misnomer as the cells do not haemolyse overnight and haemoglobinuria is not seen in half of these patients. The essential pathology is the erythrocyte mem-brane's sensitivity to complement lysis. The mechanism is due to the absence of ankyrin, which binds to complement, acting as an inactivator. This is in essence an uncontrolled complement activation with the RBC fragments as innocent bystanders.

Q83.5 What would happen if you repeated the test after heating the sera?

A83.5

There would be no lysis, as the complement is needed for the lytic process to occur.

Supplementary Question Q83.6 What indices suggest a poor prognosis for aplastic anaemia?

Supplementary Answer A83.6

WCC $< 0.4 \times 10^9/l$ for two weeks or more
Platelets $< 20 \times 10^9/l$ for two weeks or more
Reticulocytes $< 10 \times 10^9/l (< 0.1 \%)$

Supplementary Question Q83.7 What are the possible causes of death in PNH?

Supplementary Answer A83.7

Aplastic anaemia, venous thrombosis of the portal system, and infection due to leucopenia and defective leukocyte function. It may rarely progress to leukaemia.

Case 84

Q84.1 What is your subsequent management?

A84.1

This boy has status asthmaticus and one should begin an aminophylline infusion, leaving out the loading dose with i.v. hydrocortisone, and check for a pneumothorax while contacting the ITU for a possible transfer. If the $PaCO_2$ is normal, it suggests that he is becoming tired and that there is imminent respiratory arrest.

It has been agreed that many cases of asthma are underestimated and patients die because they are not admitted early. Salmeterol was originally thought to be a useful β_2-stimulant with an exo-receptor location (suggesting that it could act like the tap key of the Morse code machine). It was thus given twice daily and claimed to have added anti-inflammatory benefits. Unfortunately, clinical trials have not been so successful as *in vitro* studies. Sodium cromoglycate is still often used as a mast cell stabiliser.

Case 85

Q85.1   What has happened here?

A85.1

He has used a defence mechanism called 'intellectualisation'. Defence mechanisms are Freudian concepts, where the nature of reality has to be protected from the ego. It is a form of psychological adaptation. One cannot prove it empirically. They are subconscious and it is essential for the preservation of sanity. By its nature it is also dynamic and alters in the face of overwhelming reality. Certain forms of defence may be associated with psychopathology but not always. It is vital to understand that these mechanisms are dynamic and alter rapidly. An understanding of intellectualisation may explain some of the apparently 'illogical' reactions seen in patients during various phases of therapy.

Mature defences are seen as beneficial, since longitudinal studies show that those who exhibit them later do better in their careers. The mature defences are humour, sublimation, suppression and anticipation (which is a preparation for coming events). The term 'defence' is a concept borrowed from immunology.

Q85.2   What are the other defence mechanisms?

A85.2

These are broadly subdivided into narcissistic, immature and neurotic. Narcissistic defences are projection (e.g. a man attracted to a woman sees the woman as having a crush on him), denial (e.g. a young man who has been told that he has had a heart attack after a cocaine binge discharges himself and runs round the block), and splitting (which is sometimes associated with a borderline personality disorder). In this defence, the world is perceived as either good or bad and there is no middle ground. The realities of life are painted in shades of grey and there are few black and white situations. Such patients may describe a physician as a god or the devil on different days.

Q85.3   What are immature defences?

A85.3

Examples of these are blocking (e.g. a student who studied all night and suddenly goes blank when asked about his favourite topic), regression (e.g. one goes back to an earlier stage of development), somatisation (e.g. a headache when nervous), and introjection (e.g. a close friend of a person takes on his mannerisms when he is killed suddenly). Incidentally, introjection is a form of learning. It is not surprising to hear the mannerisms and words of your mother-in-law in your wife during arguments.

Q85.4 What are neurotic defences?

A85.4

Examples are displacement (e.g. scapegoat), repression (e.g. forgetting one's notes before an examination), isolation of affect, intellectualisation, rationalisation, reaction formation and undoing.

Q85.5 What are transference and countertransference?

A85.5

Transference is not a defence mechanism. It is considered as a form of stimulus response by learning theorists. Patients may 'transfer' thoughts or emotions regarding their significant other, or parents, to the physician. This may be pleasant or repulsive and accepted by some schools of cognitive therapy as part of therapy. If the transference is positive, he may confide his innermost thoughts to the physician. This is the reason why Hippocrates described the 'sacrosanct nature' of the patient–doctor relationship and the importance of confidentiality. The father of medicine said, 'Whatever in connection with my professional practice, or not in connection with it, I may see or hear in the lives of men which ought not to be spoken of abroad I will not divulge, as reckoning that all such should be kept secret.' A psychiatrist may not go out with his patient until two years have elapsed since the last consultation.

Countertransference is the transference of the doctor to the patient. This may be diagnosed if the physician feels that the patient has characteristics and mannerisms similar to that of his own parents, wife or sibling. These emotions may be pleasant or unpleasant, and may make an objective analysis difficult. One should refer the patient to a colleague if this is a problem. These phenomena are subconscious and dynamic and cannot be empirically proved. A failure to understand them may be a barrier to achieving a good rapport with the patient, which is essential to facilitate recovery.

Case 86

Q86.1 What is the diagnosis?

Answer 86.1

Pulmonary embolism (PE). The breathlessness is due to a ventilation–perfusion mismatch. The time course is compatible with the diagnosis.

Most orthopaedic surgeons would prefer the anticoagulation regime to be reduced prior to hip replacement to allow a relatively less bloody field. This increases the risk of embolism. The presence of pleuritic chest pain suggests that the PE is small because it has infarcted a peripheral zone.

Q86.2 How would you confirm this?

Answer 86.2

A ventilation perfusion scan will show the mismatch but angiography is the gold standard for diagnosing PE.

Q86.3 What may be seen on the CXR?

Answer 86.3

The CXR is usually normal but zones of atelectasis may be seen. After a few days, a characteristic wedge-shaped zone of infarction may be observed next to the pleura. This is known as the Hampton sign and is not seen during the acute phase of PE.

Q86.4 How would you treat this patient?

Answer 86.4

He should be started on heparin and changed to warfarin for six months. The role of thrombolysis is controversial. If the patient has a recurrence of PE despite heparin therapy, one should consider the use of a filter. If this happens, one should also carry out a thrombophilia screen. This includes protein C, protein S, antithrombin III deficiency and the presence of lupus anticoagulant.

Case 87

Q87.1 What is the diagnosis?

A87.1

Disseminated intravascular coagulation (DIC; consumption coagulopathy), either due to trauma or a Gram-negative septicaemia (in view of the emergency surgery).

Q87.2 How would you confirm this?

A87.2

Raised FDPs, blood film showing schistocytes.

Q87.3 In what other conditions can it occur?

A87.3

This can occur following the release of thromboplastic chemicals into the bloodstream following any trauma, obstetric emergencies, a retained dead foetus, metastatic cancer, acute promyelocytic leukaemia, Gram-negative sepsis, antigen–antibody reaction and myocardial infarction.

Q87.4 What is the treatment?

A87.4

Treatment of the presumed Gram-negative sepsis with antibiotics and treatment of shock must be aggressive. There must be close liaison with a haematologist and continuous monitoring. While monitoring the stability of his vital signs, give two units of FFP, fresh blood and platelets are needed. The use of heparin is controversial.

Supplementary Question Q87.5   What is unique about the DIC seen in APML (M3)?

Supplementary Answer A87.5

The DIC worsens before it improves on chemotherapy because it will not stop until nearly all the M3 cells are killed. The DIC should be managed with FFP and not heparin.

Case 88

Q88.1 What are the abnormalities?

A88.1

Very high right ventricular pressure. An increase in oxygen saturation at ventricular level, a decrease in oxygen saturation at the left ventricular level and a drop in pressure in the pulmonary artery suggest pulmonary stenosis and VSD, suggestive of Fallot's tetralogy.

Q88.2 What are the complications?

A88.2

Polycythaemia, gout, high blood viscosity, endocarditis, paradoxical emboli, syncope and arrhythmias (which may lead to death). Sometimes these patients squat to force more blood into the pulmonary circuit in an effort to increase the oxygenation of the blood. A right sided aorta occurs in 25% of cases. Operative repairs are possible. The classic repair is the Taussig–Blalock conceptualised by Helen Taussig and executed by Blalock. The Blalock shunt is usually performed on very young infants and produces a continuous murmur, representing the continuous blood flow to the pulmonary arteries. Complete surgical correction of this condition is now possible, even in the very young.

Case 89

Q89.1   What is the diagnosis?

A89.1

This patient has a cerebellar abscess which will show up readily on an MRI scan.

Case 90

Q90.1   What is the diagnosis and prognosis?

A90.1

This is classic lithium-induced hypothyroidism with hypercalcaemia and exacerbation of psoriasis. Other complications of lithium therapy include transient exacerbation of the mania paradoxically, reversible T-wave flattening, and nephrogenic diabetes insipidus.

Another drug used for manic depressive psychosis is carbamazepine, which may rarely cause bone marrow suppression. One must not stop the lithium immediately as the danger of suicide may outweigh the beneficial effects of treating the hypothyroidism. It is vital that the drug is monitored regularly. Close liaison with the psychiatrist concerned is essential in his management. The personality change may be a form of 'myxoedema psychosis'. One should take heart in the fact that Isaac Newton, the first Lucasian Professor of Physics, was said to have suffered from MDP.

Q90.2   What is the acute treatment of mania?

A90.2

It is not lithium! One may use i.v. haloperidol or a benzodiazepine.

Q90.3 *A week after discharge, he complained of headache, photophobia and vomiting. On examination, he was febrile at 39°C. Kernig's sign was positive and neurological examination was normal. An LP revealed the following:*

Opening pressure *18 cm water*
White cells *220 mm³ (78% lymphocytes)*
Protein *4 g/l*
Glucose *3 mmol/l (blood 5 mmol/l)*

He improved over the next four days. Fundoscopy revealed papilloedema and bilateral weakness of the leg. The Babinski reflex is bilaterally positive. What is the diagnosis?

A90.3

Sagittal sinus thrombosis owing to the dehydration. He should be rehydrated. MRA (magnetic resonance angiography) will confirm the diagnosis. One should liaise closely with a neurologist concerning anticoagulation, especially if there are zones of haemorrhagic cerebral infarction.

Case 91

Q91.1 *What is the diagnosis?*

A91.1

This woman has hyperthyroidism, hyperparathyroidism, and lanugo hair. Hypertrichosis lanuginosa is associated with hyperthyroidism and occult neoplasms. This will be confirmed by an undetectable TSH level and an elevated PTH level.

Autoimmune diseases hunt in packs and usually coexist. Thyrotoxicosis *per se* may also cause hypercalcaemia by bone resorption.

Supplementary Question Q91.2 *What is the MEN I syndrome?*

Supplementary Answer A91.2

The MEN I syndrome comprises neoplasms of the parathyroid, pituitary gland and pancreas. There may be occasional adrenal and thyroid involvement. Some Biblical historians have suggested that Goliath may have had the MEN I syndrome. The pituitary neoplasm may have accounted for his gigantism and his skull may have been easily because he had hyperparathyroidism which weakened his skull matrix.

Supplementary Question Q91.3   What is the MEN II syndrome?

Supplementary Answer A91.3

This comprises neoplasms of the parathyroid, medullary cell carcinoma of the thyroid and phaeochromocytoma. If this is associated with mucosal neuromas, it is termed the MEN IIb syndrome.

Case 92

Q92.1   What is the diagnosis?

A92.1

This woman has chronic lymphatic leukaemia (which accounts for 25% of all leukaemias) with associated autoimmune haemolytic anaemia. The clinical features are lymphadenopathy, hepatosplenomegaly, thrombocytopenia and anaemia. Bone marrow aspiration reveals lymphocytic replacement of the normal marrow elements with B lymphocytes comprising a quarter to nearly almost all the cell. There are immunoglobulin reduced elements in the advanced stage. Haemolytic anaemia occurs as a result of warm autoantibodies in Coombs' positive haemolysis.

This is a slowly progressive disease and responds well to chlorambucil and fludarabine.

Case 93

Q93.1   What is the pulmonary abnormality and how would you confirm this?

A93.1

The patient had a relatively normal PaO_2 before exercise, which dropped precipitously after exercise. His pH and $PaCO_2$ suggest that he is in a constant sate of hyperventilation in order to maintain his oxygen level for survival.

The transfer factor TLCO (DLCO) should be low to confirm the diagnosis, being reduced to 50% below the predicted value, which in this case will not rise with exercise. It must be remembered that the TLCO may be erroneously high in haemoptysis owing to the technique used.

Case 94

Q94.1   What is the diagnosis?

Answer 94.1

Addison's disease secondary to tuberculosis. Addison's disease is confirmed by demonstrating the absence of a rise in adrenal cortisol following an i.m. dose of ACTH. In this case, an abdominal radiograph will show the calcified adrenals. Blood glucose needs to be checked.

Q94.2 How should this be treated?

Answer 94.2

Fluid repletion with plasma expanders and normal saline, i.v. glucose if the patient is hypoglycaemic, lowering the hyperkalaemia (with continuous ECG monitoring) which may be achieved temporarily with sodium bicarbonate. Ensure that the patient is not fluid overloaded. Give i.v. hydrocortisone 100 mg stat, i.m. hydrocortisone sodium succinate 100 mg every six hours, and change over to oral steroids after 72 hours. One should liaise closely with an expert in infectious diseases because the immunosuppressive effect of steroid therapy may require a step-up in the dose of antitubercular agents. It may also be necessary to alter the period of administration to prevent the TB from flaring up.

Supplementary Question 94.3   Would your diagnosis change if the patient with an Addisonian crisis is HIV positive?

Supplementary Answer 94.3

Post-mortem examinations show that 50% of HIV positive patients have CMV adrenalitis. Paradoxically the adrenal insufficiency may worsen during the initial phase of antiretroviral treatment. This may be confirmed by testing of the adrenal reserve with an infusion of ACTH.

Case 95

Q95.1 What is the diagnosis?

A95.1

Autoimmune chronic active hepatitis (chronic lupoid hepatitis), suggested by the high titres of ANA, elevated smooth muscle antibodies with a high serum γ-globulin mainly comprising IgG, and the absence of hepatitis B antigen. It is not uncommon to have the association with high titres of measles and rubella antibodies. Anti LKM-1 antibodies may be positive and signify a more aggressive disease. Autoimmune diseases hunt in packs and this disease may be associated with the polyglandular autoimmune syndrome.

Q95.2   What is the differential diagnosis of CAH?

A95.2

This includes viral causes, alcohol, Wilson's disease and α_1-antitrypsin deficiency, and also drugs such as nitrofurantoin, isoniazid and methyldopa.

Case 96

Q96.1   What is expected on the ECG and what would you advise?

A96.1

Sinus bradycardia is a common problem with an inferior infarct. It tends to recover but, if it is persistently slow to the point of a long pause, one should pace this patient.

The jugular route is preferred as this does not contraindicate thrombolysis. The jugular route also has a more direct angle through the tricuspid valve orifice and there is much less likelihood of causing a pneumothorax.

Q96.2   What clinical pattern did he describe prior to this infarct?

A96.2

The clinical picture is highly suggestive of the subclavian steal syndrome and a neurological opinion should be sought.

Q96.3   In a normal anterior infarct, or in a small number of patients who become pacemaker-dependent, when should one pace and which mode is indicated?

A96.3

The longer a temporary wire is kept *in situ*, the greater is the risk of infection. The cut-off time is two weeks before one should pace. A normal fit patient should have a DDD system, but if the patient is in atrial fibrillation, one should use a VVI system. It must be remembered that a VVI system predisposes in time to atrial fibrillation and pacemaker syndrome, and it has greater associated morbidity. The atrial electrode may be a screw tip (which is more stable and easier to fix) or looped.

There is now a great deal of sophistication in pacemaker choice, with over thousands of permutations. The most expensive pacemaker is not always the best.

Some of the variables built into the system may cause iatrogenic pacemaker problems.

As Voltaire may be paraphrased, 'Better is the enemy of good', and it is wise to follow the American guidelines for pacemaker implants, as their actuarial studies (insurance companies) have identified the indications.

There are single-lead pacemaker systems, which have a floating sensor in the right atrium to sense the 'p' wave to allow atrioventricular synchrony, but this is not technically as effective as a lead in the atrium. The VDD system was originally designed for those operators without adequate experience in DDD pacemaker implant systems. Current evidence suggests that the floating atrial sensor is not as efficient as a conventional DDD system.

Case 97

Q97.1 What is the diagnosis?

A97.1

Familial hypokalaemic periodic paralysis, suggested by the singularly low potassium level in the absence of any other causes of hypokalaemia. This condition is common among the Chinese and the Japanese and may be associated with thyrotoxicosis.

Case 98

Q98.1 What is the diagnosis?

A98.1

Pyloric stenosis due to a neoplasm. The raised bicarbonate in the presence of a pathological urea level rules out renal destruction, as it would not be able to compensate for the vomiting and hence the loss of hydrogen ions and chloride. Sodium, HCl and potassium are lost. As hydrogen ions are lost, the blood becomes alkalotic and this effect is additive to the renal exchange of potassium and hydrogen ions.

Q98.2 What will be the pH of the urine?

A98.2

The renal reaction to persistent vomiting is to conserve sodium at the expense of potassium and hydrogen ions, hence the phenomenon of paradoxical aciduria despite an acidic plasma state.

Q98.3 Why has this patient got metabolic alkalosis?

A98.3

The reasons for metabolic alkalosis and consequent hypokalaemia are complex. He is alkalotic as he is losing hydrochloric acid from the stomach. He is also taking liquid sodium bicarbonate and diuretics. The combination of fluid loss from vomiting and diuretics is producing 'contraction alkalosis'. The alkalosis produces hypokalaemia.

Case 99

Q99.1 What is the diagnosis?

A99.1

This man has overloaded his iron stores and has reduced iron-binding capacity. He is diabetic and an elevated ALT. The diagnosis is haemo-chromatosis.

Q99.2 How else may this condition present?

A99.2

The name of bronzed diabetes was given to this patient's state as there is increase skin pigmentation. The organs affected are the liver, pancreas, heart and skin. There is an increased incidence of primary hepatoma and the condition is more common in men because women lose blood monthly during menstruation.

Q99.3 How should this patient be treated?

A99.3

Desferrioxamine, aggressive phlebotomy and diabetic control.

Supplementary Question Q99.4   What are the causes of restrictive cardiomyopathy?

Supplementary Answer A99.4

These include sarcoidosis, amyloidosis, Loeffler's endocarditis and endo-myocardial fibrosis.

Case 100

Q100.1 What is the diagnosis?

A100.1

Scurvy, as is supported by his lifestyle and diet. His gynaecomastia is due to marijuana, which is an antiandrogen. The bleeding is due to weak vessels.

The differential diagnosis of the purpura is amyloidosis, Cushing's syndrome and a qualitative platelet defect (such as the Bernard–Soulier syndrome, in which there are functionally defective giant platelets). Other causes are drug induced purpura, senile purpura, Henoch–Schoenlein purpura, dysproteinaemia, Ehlers–Danlos syndrome and pseudoxanthoma elasticum.

Q100.2 What else should be assessed?

A100.2

The possibility of osteomalacia must be borne in mind. One should look for the biochemical profile of a raised serum alkaline phosphatase and low serum calcium, which may require adequate dietary support.

Q100.3 One week after hospitalisation he demonstrated a relatively normal PT but a prolonged PTT. What has happened?

A100.3

The combination of a poor diet in hospital with antibiotic therapy has compromised the absorption of vitamin K and prolonged the PTT. This should be corrected with FFP and subcutaneous vitamin K.

Case 101

Q101.1 What are the possible diagnoses?

A101.1

This is compatible with shock (low BP) before hypercapnoea developed owing to the bleeding ulcer. This should be endoscoped with a simultaneous infusion of colloid and blood. There is a good possibility that an endoscopic heater tip probe could seal the ulcer point. A sentinel bleeding point, if identified, can be controlled accurately.

The low PaO_2 and the normal $PaCO_2$ make this a type 1 respiratory failure, which is seen frequently in acute asthmatic attacks as the patient is becoming exhausted. Many such patients are also dehydrated and should be admitted and treated aggressively.

Case 102

Q102.1 What is the diagnosis?

Answer 102.1

Acute thoracic dissection of the aorta with occlusion of the arteries of the cord. The pulses may be unequal in both arms and, if it dissects back-wards, there may be an inferior infarction, a renal infarction (relatively rare) and hemiplegia, which may be a consequence of involvement of the carotid artery. This catastrophic cystic medial tear is painless in 10-20% of cases. Some present with hypertension, which must be con-trolled. An early diastolic murmur may also be detectable if the aortic valve is torn.

Q102.2 How would you diagnose it?

Answer 102.2

CXR for a widened mediastinum or a CT scan of the thorax, but the simplest method is by TOE, which gives an excellent view of an aortic dissection, and aids surgical planning. In this particular case, TOE is contraindicated in view of the dysphagia because it may cause perfora-tion of the oesophagus.

Case 103

Q103.1 What is the diagnosis and how will you confirm this?

A103.1

This likely to be an ostium secundum ASD with Ebstein's anomaly with the Wolff–Parkinson–White syndrome. This can be diagnosed by echo-cardiography, which will show atrialisation of a large part of the right ventricle. A large part of the output is therefore dependent on right atrial contraction. The palpitations are due to tachyarrhythmias, which will be detected by Holter monitoring. With the high pressure from the Epstein's anomaly, there will be a shunt through an ASD of a PFO, which an agitated saline echo will demonstrate. TOE will allow a better visualisation of the anatomy.

Q103.2 How would you treat the palpitations?

A103.2

This patient has palpitations which may be due to the Wolff–Parkinson–

White syndrome. This is a congenital condition caused by an abnormal myocardial connection between the atrium and the ventricle. If the QRS is upright in V1, this is a type A syndrome and if it is inverted, it is type B. Digoxin and verapamil are contraindicated in the Wolff–Parkinson–White syndrome. Digoxin may paradoxically improve conduction down the abnormal pathway. If the patient is symptomatic, treatment should be by radiofrequency ablation of the abnormal pathway. Symptomatic patients may also be treated with class Ia, Ic and III drugs if ablation is unsuccessful or refused.

Case 104

Q104.1 What is the most likely diagnosis?

A104.1

He has contracted Creutzfeld–Jakob (CJD) disease from infected pituitary gland extracts.

Prions do not have DNA and may be transmitted from one species to another. Recent experiments have fulfilled parts of Koch's postulates and produced a form of bovine spongiform encephalopathy in primates and proved that it is capable of crossing the species barrier. The other prion diseases are kuru, familial fatal insomnia, Gerstmann–Straussler–Scheinker disease and scrapie. CJD has also been associated with corneal transplants and stereotaxic needles.

A differential diagnosis would be chronic subdural haematoma suggested by the history of horse riding, but this is excluded by the CT scan. Another possibility is normal pressure hydrocephalus, which is the triad of ataxia, dementia and urinary incontinence.

Q104.2 What is the gold standard for the diagnosis of this disease?

A104.2

Unfortunately the only way to diagnose this with any accuracy is by brain biopsy or at post-mortem. Recent publications suggest that there may be a new test for CJD based on immunoassay of 14-3-3 protein in the CSF. This test promises high sensitivity and specificity. 'Blind' testing of samples of CSF fluid from patients with the classic and 'new variant CJD' have shown some promising results. There is, as yet, no specific test is available for the 'new variant disease'.

Case 105

Q105.1 What is the diagnosis?

A105.1

This woman has bulimia. She induces vomiting by purgative abuse, which accounts for the massive loss of potassium from the large gut. Hypokalaemic alkalosis and normal renal function may also be seen in long-term diuretic abuse.

Bulimia rarely affects men, in whom the prognosis is poorer. Bulimia occurs due to the distortion of a person's body image. She should be referred for psychiatric management and cognitive psychotherapy. Potassium repletion is critical and the dangers of arrhythmias associated with chronic hypokalaemia should be explained.

Q105.2   What other states may present with such a biochemical profile?

A105.2

Hypokalaemic alkalosis may also be seen in steroid therapy, Cushing's disease, Conn's syndrome (due to excess potassium loss either from an adrenal adenoma or bilateral adrenal hyperplasia) and excess carbenoxolone prescribed as ulcer therapy.

Case 106

Q106.1 What is the diagnosis?

A106.1

Acute vitamin A intoxication with benign intracranial hypertension, which will be confirmed by a serum assay for vitamin A. Seals have a disproportionate amount of fat in their liver, which is why the Eskimo tribe avoid it. Some polar explorers have reported desquamation of the soles of their feet, clubbing, coarse sparse hair, anaemia and nausea. Benign intracranial hypertension may also be associated with outdated tetracycline use.

Case 107

Q107.1 What is the likely diagnosis?

A107.1

Thrombotic thrombocytopenic purpura (TTP). There is no evidence of DIC. TTP is caused by activation of the platelets, resulting in agglutination in vital organs and usually presents with fever, neurological features, renal failure, microangiopathic haemolytic anaemia (MAHA) and thrombocytopenia. There is an increased incidence in the six months following pregnancy.

The differential diagnosis includes pre-eclampsia, which must be excluded, as this can still occur after the delivery of the foetus. The worst case senario of this condition is HELP syndrome, which is characterised by the accumulation of fluid in the liver (elevating the hepatic enzymes), thrombocytopenia, haemolysis and toxaemia. The patient may complain of right upper quadrant pain, blurring of vision and confusion. Despite the accumulation of fluid, there is no dependent oedema.

Q107.2 What is the treatment?

A107.2

Infusion of FFP replaces the missing factor that inhibits platelet agglutination. In some patients, there are circulating factors which activate platelets. These patients benefit from plasmapharesis. The efficiency of prostacyclin and heparin is not proved, and platelet infusion should be avoided as it will cause further aggrevation.

Case 108

Q108.1 What is the diagnosis and how should this be managed?

A108.1

This man has AIDS with PCP and thrombocytopenia. Kaposi's sarcoma is more common with homosexuals. The sputum should be Gram-stained, and Grocott (silver) stained for PCP, and Ziehl–Nielsen stained for acid-fast bacilli. One should remember that AIDS patients may have atypical mycobacterial infection and may be infected by several organisms simultaneously. Routine culture for mycobacteria should be carried out. Nebulised hypertonic saline should be administered in those in whom the sputum is scanty. Broncho-alveolar lavage with transbronchial biopsy is the gold standard for diagnosis. A practical approach is to treat it empirically and only perform bronchoscopy if the patient is not improving.

If the diagnosis of PCP is confirmed, therapy should be started with high-dose cotrimoxazole.

Q108.2 Why is he so rigid?

A108.2

It is possible that the compound he injected contained MPTP, which is a contaminant in illicitly-produced heroin. It is a toxin which targets the substantia nigra and destroys it, producing clinical parkinsonism. These respond to dopamine. Experiments with rats pretreated with selegeline and injected with MPTP show that they do not develop substantia nigra destruction. This encourages its use in early Parkinson's disease. The DATATOP study suggested that selegeline may retard the deteriorative velocity of the parkinsonism, but recent data suggest that it may reduce the lifespan of the participants. Whether to give selegeline or not is a contentious area at present, but the tragedy of the frozen addicts has given us an insight into this ailment.

Q108.3   A few months after starting antiretroviral therapy, he complained of shooting pains and weakness on climbing stairs. Investigations: Hb 8 g/l, WCC 3 × 10⁹/l, platelets 100 × 10⁹, MCV 94 fl and CPK 655 IU/l. What is the diagnosis?

A108.3

Zidovudine-induced proximal myopathy and induced bone marrow suppression.

Supplementary Question Q108.4   How would you treat PCP?

Supplementary Answer A108.4

One should use trimethoprim and sulphamethoxazole empirically in the acute phase. The CXR is usually abnormal but may be normal. If he is allergic to these two drugs, use pentamidine i.v. It must be borne in mind that pentamidine is used experimentally to produce a rat model of diabetes, so pancreatitis and IDDM must be anticipated and treated. Aerosolised pentamidine and dapsone may be used as prophylaxis.

There is persuasive evidence that steroids may be used in PCP, although this appears counterintuitive. Steroids reduce the amount of interstitial disease and reduce the hypoxia. The diagnosis of PCP is confirmed by broncho-alveolar lavage.

Case 109

Q109.1   What is the diagnosis?

Answer 109.1

Acute intermittent porphyria. Attacks usually occur in the third and fourth decades. She should stop using the barbiturate and the oral contraceptives. This is inherited as an autosomal dominant trait. One of the presentations is abdominal pain without guarding, which explains the laparotomy.

The other components of this disease (which frequently precede the acute episode) are leucocytosis, fever, gastric dilatation, motor peripheral neuropathy, ophthalmoplegia, optic atrophy, facial palsy, and emotional and psychiatric disturbance. Vagal neuropathy may cause sinus tachycardia and attacks may be precipitated by barbiturates, alcohol, sulphonamides, griseofulvin, oestrogens and a wide range of lipid-soluble drugs.

Q109.2 How would you confirm the diagnosis?

Answer 109.2

There is excessive δ-aminolaevulinic acid (ALA) and porphobilinogen (PBG) in the urine. In acute intermittent porphyria there is a problem with the enzyme (uroporphyrinogen I synthetase) which catalyses the conversion of PBG to uroporphyrinogen I. In lead poisoning, which is the major differential diagnosis, as it may also cause encephalopathy and peripheral neuropathy. There is interference with the enzyme ALA dehydrase, which raises the δ-ALA dehydrase (with normal PBG), and inhibition of the enzyme ferrochelatase, causing an additional rise in protoporphyrin IX.

A field test for urinary PBG is to add 2 ml of Ehrlich's aldehyde to 2 mo of the 'suspect' urine. A pink colour indicates the presence of either urobilinogen or PBG. If the pink colour remains in the top layer after the addition of 4 ml of chloroform, the urine contains an excess of PBG.

Q109.3 How would you manage her?

Answer 109.3

This is predominantly supportive in the acute phase. A high carbo-hydrate diet will indirectly reduce porphyrin production. An opioid like pethidine or morphine may be given for pain relief, valium may be prescribed for insomnia, and a haematin infusion may be used. The patient should also be counselled to avoid precipitating factors such as drugs and alcohol.

Case 110

Q110.1 What is the diagnosis?

A110.1

VSD with Eisenmenger syndrome. The drop in saturation in the left ventricle suggests that some deoxygenated blood is flowing into the right ventricle from the left ventricle.

Case 111

Q111.1   What is the diagnosis?

A111.1

Insulinoma (but a C peptide assay must be performed to rule out factitious hypoglycaemia because her son is a diabetic)

Q111.2   What investigations would you perform?

A111.2

The aim is to locate the source of the neoplasm: CT scanning (usually does not locate the tumour because of its minute size); MRI of the abdomen; selective arteriography (coeliac axis angiography) may demonstrate tumour blush. One may also perform percutaneous transhepatic catheterisation of the splenic and portal veins with sampling for insulin, and ultrasound scanning of the pancreatic head and duodenal wall using a probe mounted on an endoscope.

Another possible investigation involves a direct ultrasound probe scan in direct contact with the pancreas during exploratory laparotomy and inspection of the pancreas. The C peptide suppression test measures C peptide during hypoglycaemia induced by purified insulin. Failure to suppress C peptide suggests an autonomous tumour inappropriately producing insulin.

Q111.3   What is the definitive treatment?

A111.3

Surgical resection of the insulinoma.

Case 112

Q112.1   What is the likely diagnosis?

A112.1

This woman has hyperosmolar hyperglycaemic coma, precipitated by a urinary tract infection. The glucose level was further elevated by Lucozade, which is a sugar-rich drink made famous by an excellent advertisement by one of Britain's greatest athletes and considered to be a panacea by some Afro-Caribbean groups. HONK is more common in the elderly. In this condition the insulin resistance of ketoacidosis is absent.

Q112.2 What are the essential investigations?

A112.2

Blood glucose is usually above 35 mmol/l in HONK. Urine and blood cultures, an ECG and a CKMB estimation should be carried out (as it may sometimes be precipitated by a myocardial infarction). There is pseudohyponatraemia due to the high glucose. Acidosis is absent as there is no switch to ketone metabolism.

Q112.3 How would you treat this condition?

A112.3

Pass a nasogastric tube immediately as there may be gastroparesis. This may be associated with pulmonary aspiration. The mainstay of therapy is still normal saline to correct the fluid deficit. Infuse insulin but beware of the sudden plummeting glucose level, as these patients are extremely sensitive to insulin. Hypotonic saline should not be administered except in exceptional circumstances. A few hours of hypernatraemia is less detrimental to the brain than sudden hyponatraemia.

Potassium repletion may be necessary. Heparin prophylaxis should be given as there is a risk of deep vein thrombosis. Long-term insulin may not be needed and the primary infection should be treated.

Q112.4 How would you analyse hyponatraemia?

A112.4

One should first assess the patient to see if she is dry and euvolaemic. If there is oedema, the patient has nephrotic syndrome, cirrhosis or congestive cardiac failure.

If the patient is hypovolaemic, consider the possibility of Addison's disease, salt-losing nephritis, the overuse of diuretics, vomiting and diarrhoea.

If the patient is euvolaemic, consider pseudohyponatraemia, SIADH, acute water intoxication or the rare hyporeninaemic hypoaldosteronism. The causes of pseudohyponatraemia includes elevated levels of glucose, lipids, triglycerides and proteins.

Case 113

Q113.1 What has occurred?

A113.1

A leucoerythroblastic blood film (the blasts are the juvenile red and white cells) due to TB, which should recover with successful therapy.

Q113.2 How is this confirmed?

A113.2

Bone marrow aspiration.

Q113.3 What other conditions may cause this?

A113.3

Any condition which causes of the marrow and pushes out the normal younger cells may cause this picture, e.g. CML, secondaries from breast, bronchus, stomach or prostate, multiple myeloma and polycythaemia rubra vera.

Case 114

Q114.1 What is the diagnosis?

A114.1

This is extrinsic allergic alveolitis, which develops 4–8 hours after inhaling spores of *Micropolyspora faeni*. This is a Type III and IV allergic reaction (Coomb and Gell classification) or an Arthus reaction dependent on the circulating antibody (not IgE) and inhaled antigen locking together, forming a complex which affects the lung. The disease is not confined to farmers, and may be seen in gypsies who live rough in old damp buildings that harbour the culprit spore.

The characteristic history is an improvement in hospital. The symptoms recur when these patients return home.

Q114.2 What pattern of lung function abnormalities may be deduced?

A114.2

There is a restrictive pattern of lung function, hypoxia and reduced gas transfer.

The low gas transfer suggests a lung parenchymal pathology. Repeated exposures lead to granulomatous changes with diffuse pulmonary fibrosis. On auscultation, crackles may be heard but often not as prominently as in crytogenic fibrosing alveolitis. Clubbing may occur in the later stages of fibrosis. Unlike CFA, the alterations in the lungs are more prominent in the upper zones.

Q114.3 What is the treatment?

A114.3

Treatment in the acute phase is prednisolone. Long-term therapy involves avoidance of sites where these moulds grow, or, if it is an occupational hazard, these patients should keep away from mouldy hay (spores). If this is impossible, consider using a respirator when handling hay.

Q114.4 How do you analyse interstitial lung disease (ILD)?

A114.4

A non-occupational cause of ILD is idiopathic fibrosing alveolitis. This subgroup has soft crackles and 30% are ANA positive. The other group comprises those subject to occupational hazards caused by either organic or inorganic dust.

ILD associated with organic dust is farmer's lung, in which the pre-cipitin test is positive. The diseases involving the interstitium and caused by inorganic dust are coal miner's pneumoconiosis, asbestosis, silicosis, berylliosis and Caplan's syndrome. Silicosis is associated with sandblasting and has an 'egg shell' calcific X-ray appearance. Silicosis may coexist with TB, in which case it is called silicotuberculosis.

Asbestosis may progress to mesothelioma but the most commonly associated neoplasms are adenocarcinoma or squamous cell carcinoma.

Supplementary Question Q114.5   What are the broncho-alveolar lavage findings in farmer's lung?

Supplementary Answer A114.5

Broncho-alveolar lavage findings are elevated lymphocytes (like sarcoid-osis), cf. in CFA, where neutrophils are raised.

Supplementary Question Q114.6   What are the types of extrinsic allergic alveolitis?

Supplementary Answer A114.6

These are farmer's lung, where the source of the antigen is mouldy hay, straw or grain and the antigen may be *Micropolyspora faeni* or *Thermo-actinomyces vulgaris*. It may also be seen in bird fanciers, where the source of the antigen is avian serum. There is a rare form associated with sugar cane called bagassosis, caused by *Thermoactinomyces sacchari*. A new form of occupational lung disease in this category has been associated with polyurethane foam manufacturers, caused by diisocyanates. Where the antigen has been identified, serological tests are available to detect the precipitating IgG antibody in the blood. However, exposed people may have the antibody without the disease.

Case 115

Q115.1   What is the diagnosis?

Answer 115.1

The syndrome of inappropriate antidiuretic hormone (SIADH) secretion due to carbamazepine. The urine sodium concentration is raised. A rapid confirmatory test is urinary osmolality, which would be very high.

Q115.2   What is the treatment?

Answer 115.2

Treat the fit with diazepam and use an alternative to carbamazepine after stopping it. If the fitting recurs, give phenytoin with ECG monitoring. Restrict fluids and do not use hypertonic saline because rapid normal-isation of the sodium may cause central pontine myelinolysis. If simple cessation of carbamazepine does not correct the situation, one should seek other causes of SIADH: head injury (CT scan will be normal in this case), cancer of bronchus, chlorpropamide, thiazides and hypothyroid-ism all stimulate vasopressin release. Remember that very high levels of glucose or triglycerides may cause pseudohyponatraemia. If fluid restric-tion fails, demeclocycline or lithium, which produces a reversible form of diabetes insipidus, may help SIADH.

Case 116

Q116.1   What is the differential diagnosis?

A116.1

The high urinary catecholamine level suggests either a rebound phenomenon from missing his regular antihypertensive medication or phaeochromocytoma. The profile fits the picture of clonidine with-drawal. Clonidine is a centrally acting presynaptic α_2-adrenergic agonist, which increases the storage of sympathomimetic neurotransmitters in the terminal nerve endings by stimulating the α_2-inhibitory receptors. If the drug is suddenly withdrawn, stored amines are released producing a phaeochromocytoma-like syndrome and their urinary excretion is in-creased. A transdermal formulation has been designed to reduce side effects.

Q116.2 How should he be treated?

A116.2

The acute therapy is the reintroduction of clonidine, as this will reverse the symptoms and rapidly lower the BP. Labetalol (which has α- and β-blocking properties) can be given parenterally.

Supplementary Question Q116.3 What is clonidine?

Supplementary Answer A116.3

This is a centrally acting presynaptic α_2-agonist. It may be used transdermally to reduce the side effects. The chronic use of this drug has been shown to reduce left ventricular hypertrophy. The side effects include sedation, insomnia, dry mouth, dizziness and bradycardia. Sudden withdrawal may produce a syndrome such as the one described above.

Case 117

Q117.1 What is the diagnosis?

RAA

A117.1

Conn's syndrome (primary hyperaldosteronism), which will be confirmed by a raised aldosterone level without an associated elevation of renin. This saline provocation test suggests excess mineralocorticoid presence because it induces hypokalaemia but retains salt.

Q117.2 What are the other causes of polyuria?

A117.2

Hypokalaemia *per se* as well as hypercalcaemia from cancer of the bronchus (with lytic bone deposits) may cause renal tubular damage. If the hypercalcaemia is due to lung cancer, it would suggest an oat cell tumour that produces PTH.

Case 118

Q118.1 What is the diagnosis?

A118.1

Turner's syndrome (46XO) or pure gonadal dysgenesis. This is a form of hypergonadotrophic hypogonadism.

Q118.2 How is this confirmed?

A118.2

Karyotyping will confirm the diagnosis by demonstrating an XO chromosomal abnormality, an XX/XO mosaic combination or a permutation of XO/XXX, XO, XXX/XX mosaicism, or structural abnormalities of the X chromosome (e.g. 46 isochromosome Xq–, Xp–).

Turner's syndrome has a frequency of 1:5000 live births. Characteristically, streak ovaries are present. The clinical features include a short stature with a low hairline, infertility and webbing of the neck. Other features include cystic hygroma, peripheral lymphoedema at birth and a preductal form of coarctation of the aorta.

There is a mental retardation in 12% of these patients.

Supplementary Question Q118.3 What is mosaicism?

Supplementary Answer A118.3

These are mitotic errors (e.g. uneven distribution of chromosomes in somatic daughter cells or cleavage of the fertilised ovum) during early development, resulting in more than one population of cells in one individual. It affects the sex chromosomes more often than the autosomal chromosomes.

Supplementary Question Q118.4   What is Noonan's syndrome?

Supplementary Answer A118.4

This is the Turner phenotype with normal 46XX (or 46XY) affecting both sexes. There is normal fertility and there is also an increased likelihood of right sided cardiac lesions, cf. Turner's syndrome involves the left side (such as ASD, VSD, AS and coarctation of the aorta).

Case 119

Q119.1 What is the most likely diagnosis?

A119.1

Von Willebrand's disease, which is inherited as an autosomal dominant trait.

Q119.2 What is the abnormality in this disorder?

A119.2

The essential disorder is an abnormal platelet adhesion in association with low Factor VIII activity. There is also defective platelet aggregation with ristocetin, which is an antibiotic that was removed from the market because of thrombocytopenia, as it induces platelet aggregation in normal platelet-rich plasma. This, however, does not happen in patients with the severe form of von Willebrand's disease. In the majority of patients, the aggregation is positive to other agents, e.g. ADP, collagen, thrombin and adrenaline. Low levels of von Willebrand factor can occur.

Q119.3 How would you treat this disorder?

A119.3

The bleeding episodes are treated with intermediate-purity Factor VIII concentrates that contain von Willebrand factor and Factor VIII, or with DDAVP. Factor VIII infusions may cause sustained and delayed increases of Factor VIII clotting activity. This is because the infused von Willebrand factor in the Factor VIII preparation prolongs the survival of the patient's own Factor VIII. Bleeding from the orifices may be treated by tranexamic acid or aminocaproic acid.

Case 120

Q120.1 What is the diagnosis?

A120.1

Emphysema due to α_1-antitrypsin deficiency. Pulmonary emphysema is usually associated with smokers. α_1-Antitrypsin is a glycoprotein and essentially a protease inhibitor which controls the multiple inflammatory cascades such as C1 inhibitor and antithrombin. α_1-Antitrypsin is produced in the liver and comprises 90% of the serum α_1-globulin visualised in electrophoresis. The gene is located on chromosome 14.

Q120.2 What are the genetic variations of this disorder?

A120.2

These are characterised by their electophoretic mobilities as medium (M), slow (S) or very slow (Z). The normal genotype is PiMM, the homozygote for Z is PiZZ. The heterozygotes are PiMZ and PiSZ. The S and Z variants are due to a single amino acid replacement of glutamic acid at positions 264 and 342 of the polypeptides respectively. This replacement results in decreased synthesis and secretion of the normal protease inhibitor as forms about 60% of that produced normally by M, while the Z variety only represents 15%. The majority of patients with clinical disease have the PiZZ phenotype.

α_1-Antitrypsin deficiency is inherited as an autosomal dominant condition and one out of 11 of northern Europeans carry this deficiency gene.

Q120.3 What other clinical manifestations may this patient have?

A120.3

Approximately 10–15% of these patients will develop cirrhosis after the age of 50 years and approximately 5% of patients will die of liver disease. There is no treatment apart from dealing with the complications of liver disease. Patients with liver failure should be considered for transplantation. They should be asked to stop smoking.

Case 121

Q121.1 What is the diagnosis?

Answer 121.1

Fish bone perforation of the oesophagus, producing mediastinal gas and pleural effusion (which may be of blood or food). Mediastinal widening is diagnostic of a haematoma. The radiograph may localise the site of perforation (but beware that a calcified hyoid bone may simulate a foreign body). A gastrograffin examination will demonstrate the tear. Serial CT scans or MRI may show the exact location of the fishbone spearing the gullet. This may aid surgical planning if necessary.

Q121.2 What is the therapy?

Answer 121.2

The patient should not be fed orally, and blood should be grouped and cross-matched. One should begin i.v. therapy against Gram-negative organisms, e.g. ampicillin, metronidazole and ampicillin. The case should be discussed with a surgeon as a large tear requires repair, but a small one may heal with masterful inactivity. An iatrogenic cause of perforation is oesophageal instrumentation.

Q121.3 What is a 'café' coronary?

Answer 121.3

This is the sudden occlusion of the upper airway with food, classically in a loquacious wine drinker, which has nothing to do with a heart attack. Experiments with beagles (suggesting that the application of a relatively mild force can extrude meat stuck in the upper airway) led to defining the Heimleich manoeuvre. This involves a backward and upward thrust of the locked fist from below the xiphisternum as one stands behind the patient. If this fails to expel the food, an emergency transverse cut must be made below the cricoid cartilage (incised at 90% to avoid severing the vocal cords) followed by the insertion of a hollow tube, such as a biro shaft, to allow respiration. This manoeuvre may be necessary as the event can occur miles from the nearest medical facility before a proper airway can be surgically crafted. Sometimes a piece of steak is stuck in the gullet and may be removed by forceps by an ENT surgeon in the appropriate setting. An attempt to remove the occluding bolus manually via the mouth may push it deeper.

Case 122

Question Q122.1 What is the diagnosis?

A122.1

This patient has aortic regurgitation due to relapsing polychondritis. The severity of the regurgitation may be assessed by the diastolic pressure (the basis of the water hammer pulse). The clinical picture suggests that the architectural changes are unlikely to be reversed by valve replacement. A left ventricular end diastolic pressure (LVEDP) greater than 20 mmHg suggests impairment of the left ventricle, which is likely to be irreversible. This is likely to be unchanged after valve replacement when an M mode echo gives an end diastolic pressure exceeding 55 mmHg.

Q122.2 When should one operate in endocarditis?

A122.2

It is an emergency situation when there is LVF with mitral regurgitation and sudden acute aortic regurgitation or if a large mobile endocardial vegetation poses a risk to embolisation.

Supplementary Question Q122.3 When should one operate in aortic regurgitation?

Supplementary Answer A122.3

There are no hard and fast rules for this. Many patients may be apparently well for many years in spite of torrential aortic regurgitation. In order to operate, one must have indicators suggesting worsening severity, such as a collapsing pulse, endocarditis or dyspnoea.

There is a 5% risk of operative mortality.

One should perform an echo cardiogram to look for the end systolic dimension and an increased end diastolic value, and assess the LV function and the ejection fraction.

The guiding principle should be to operate before there are irreversible architectural changes. They are generally irreversible if there is dyspnoea.

Supplementary Question Q122.4   What are some of the causes of aortic regurgitation?

Supplementary Answer A122.4

Rheumatic heart disease, SBE, ankylosing spondylitis, Marfan's syndrome, Ehlers–Danlos syndrome, Hurler's syndrome, relapsing polychondritis and dissecting aortic aneurysm.

Case 123

Q123.1   What is the diagnosis?

A123.1

Multiple myeloma. The combination of elevated urate, low albumin (in the face of normal liver function) and hypercalcaemia suggest myeloma. The lipids may fall if there is hypoalbuminaemia. A raised urate may accompany renal damage or myeloma. In this case the renal function deduced from the plasma creatinine was normal.

Q123.2   How would you confirm this?

A123.2

There may be rouleaux in the peripheral smear. Bence–Jones protein in the urine, a monoclonal band on electrophoresis, bone marrow aspiration and the skull X-ray changes are some of the diagnostic criteria.

Q123.3   What is the prognosis?

A123.3

Presenting features comprising renal failure and severe anaemia are some of the poor prognostic indicators, with 50% of such patients dying within nine months. If this patient is taken as a representative group, the median survival is two years.

Q123.4 What are the bad prognostic indicators of myeloma?

A123.4

They are:

Serum β_2-microglobulin	$> 5\,mg/l$
Haemoglobin	$< 7.6\,g/dl$
Serum urea	$> 13\,mmol/l$
Bence Jones proteinurea	$> 2\,g/l$
Serum albumin	$> 30\,g/l$

Case 124

Q124.1 What is the diagnosis?

A124.1

Cushing's syndrome, as suggested by the hypokalaemic alkalosis, polycythaemia and diabetes mellitus. One should consider an ectopic ACTH source.

Q124.2 What investigations would you perform?

A124.2

CT scan of the adrenals, circadian study for cortisol, dexamethasone suppression test, insulin tolerance test, urinary free cortisol, chest and skull X-ray examination.

Q124.3 What is a flat glucose tolerance curve?

A124.3

The level of glucose fails to rise normally and remains relative low throughout. This may be seen in normal individuals, hypopituitarism, Addison's disease and malabsoptive conditions.

Case 125

Q125.1 What is the diagnosis?

A125.1

Sideroblastic anaemia due to antituberculous therapy.

Q125.2 How would you classify this disorder?

A125.2

Sideroblastic anaemia may be hereditary. This hereditary form usually occurs in males but is transmitted by females. The acquired forms may be due to myelodysplasia or secondary to other malignant diseases of the marrow, such as myeloid leukaemia or myeloma. It may also be due to drugs such as alcohol, lead, and the antituberculous agents such as isoniazid and cycloserine. Benign conditions associated with sideroblastic anaemia are haemolytic anaemia, megaloblastic anaemia and malabsorption.

Case 126

Q126.1 What is the diagnosis?

Answer 126.1

This man is being poisoned with rat poison (warfarin) and this suspicion warrants a duty to inform the police who, in turn, have a duty to protect him (the tragedy of the Tarasof cases I and II clearly illustrates the danger of not doing so). He should be treated with injectable vitamin K.

Case 127

Q127.1 What is the diagnosis?

A127.1

Familial hypercholesterolaemia

Q127.2 What treatment should be advised?

A127.2

A low saturated fat diet, cholestyramine and a HMG CoA reductase inhibitor such as pravastatin or simvastatin.

Q127.3 What other test may you perform?

A127.3

A 24-hour ST segment analysis to scan for intermittent ST elevation will rule out Prinzmetal's angina. The ST elevation indicates sub-epicardial injury compared with ST depression, which indicates sub-endocardial injury. Variant angina carries a poor prognosis and should be further investigated.

Q127.4   What if he complained of a band-like pain over the left side of his chest, haematuria and impotence?

A127.4

This is highly suggestive of schistosomiasis causing radicular pain, lethargy and impotence. The wells of Jericho were contaminated with this parasite. This is why historians speculated the desertion of the city long after Joshua conquered it.

The lethargy probably explains why the walls were not built well.

Case 128

Q128.1   What is the most likely diagnosis?

A128.1

Congenital adrenal hyperplasia due to 21-hydroxylase deficiency. There is salt wasting (which is not seen in the more severe disease of 11-β-hydroxylase deficiency). The blockage is in the conversion of 17-α-hydroxyprogesterone to 11-deoxycortisol. The lack of this metabolic conversion step sets the entire system into hyperdrive, which produces a weak androgenic metabolite in vast quantities and masculinises the child. This feedback loop overdrive is prevented by the replacement of glucocorticoids.

Q128.2   How would you confirm it?

A128.2

Serum 17-α-hydroxyprogesterone level, urinary 24-hour pregnanetriol and morning plasma ACTH estimation.

Case 129

Q129.1   What is the diagnosis?

A129.1

Hyperparathyroidism resulting in a duodenal ulcer, which has caused iron deficiency anaemia. The development of haematuria and *E. coli* infection with stones is very common in von Recklinghausen's disease.

This disease is remembered by the litany, abdominal moans, bones and psychic groans.

Hypermagnesaemia is found in some of these patients; it returns to normal with adequate therapy. The parathyroid adenoma should be removed. An IVP, an endoscopy to search for the bleeding ulcer, and the urea breath test for *Helicobacter pylori* should also be performed. X-ray examination of the hands may demonstrate characteristic changes and there may be brown tumours.

Q129.2 How will you confirm and treat this disease?

A129.2

A supersensitive assay for PTH can be performed to confirm this. Differential scanning after simultaneous radiothallium and technetium administration may be performed preoperatively. The principle of surgery is the resection of all three glands, leaving one either *in situ* or transplanted subcutaneously. It is practical to implant superficially, to allow surgical extirpation should the symptoms of hypercalcaemia recur.

Case 130

Q130.1 What is the diagnosis?

Answer 130.1

Carbon monoxide poisoning. A COHb should be done stat. This simulates hypoglycaemia, which is readily ruled out by BM testing. The carbon monoxide is produced as a consequence of incomplete combustion of fuel in a heater.

Q130.2 What is the treatment?

Answer 130.2

Airway management (because they are semi-comatose). The pulse oximeter may be misleadingly normal, despite the presence of tissue hypoxia. Hyperbaric oxygen is a logical choice, although transfer to a hyperbaric chamber is controversial. A 12-lead ECG may show evidence of coronary ischaemia in CO poisoning. Fire victims who have had prolonged exposure to smoke have been known to die from myocardial infarction. Their post-mortems have demonstrated patent coronary arteries, suggesting that the cause of death was due to carbon monoxide poisoning *per se*.

Smokers have a CO level of 10% and toxicity occurs beyond 25%. CPR may be needed and vigilant rapid therapy for dysrhythmia must be available. Cardiogenic shock with metabolic acidosis is of vital importance and this is an urgent indication for referral to an ITU for ventilatory support. Remember that a pulse oximeter is useless and that an ABG estimation is crucial. 100% O_2 should be administered in all cases.

Supplementary Question 130.3 What is the difference between carbon monoxide poisoning and oxygen binding to Hb?

Supplementary Answer 130.3

CO has an infinity for haemoglobin that is 240 times greater than oxygen. The partial pressure of CO in blood is nearly zero. Oxygen is bound to Hb differently. Each Hb molecule can carry four oxygen molecules, of which the binding sites have varying affinities for O_2. The affinity for oxygen alters with either the loaded or the postloaded state of the haemoglobin.

Case 131

Q131.1 What is the initial diagnosis?

A131.1

PDA with pulmonary hypertension and mild pulmonary incompetence. This is the PDA Eisenmenger scenario. Once the Eisenmenger complex develops, closure is contraindicated.

Case 132

Q132.1 What is the diagnosis?

A132.1

Carcinoma of the bronchus with paraneoplastic cerebellar degeneration (oat cell carcinoma tends to produce ADH and squamous cell carcinoma may produce PTH, but there is no clear distinction between the two). In SIADH, the urinary sodium is high. Neoplastic cells undergo numerous evolutionary alterations during their natural course, which explains their resistance and unpredictability during therapy.

Supplementary Question Q132.2   What are the other neurological paraneoplastic syndromes?

Supplementary Answer A132.2

These include limbic encephalitis, which may produce amnesia, hallu-
cinations and epilepsy. Other features include brain stem encephalitis,
cord disease, degeneration of the dorsal root ganglia and degeneration of
the anterior horn cells. The treatment of paraneoplastic CNS degeneration is unsatisfactory. Removal of the primary neoplasm may be
followed by improvement.

Case 133

Q133.1 What is the diagnosis?

Answer 133.1

He has the 'bends'. One treats this with fluid expansion and transfer to a
hyperbaric chamber in an aircraft that can negotiate low altitudes (less
than 500 ft). He should be brought down to sea level immediately. Do
not give Entonox (laughing gas) as this will diffuse to coalesce with the
air bubbles, making them larger. The rationale of therapy is to re-
compress the bubbles in a high-pressure chamber. Ideally, road transfer
is best. This is a common ailment in pearl divers.

Q133.2 If they had eaten the wildfowl, what complications would there have been?

Answer 133.2

None as the gut enzymes would have detoxified the curare. D-Tubo-
curarine is the prototype non-depolarising neuromuscular blocker. The
other agents in this group are doxacurium, pancuronium, vecuronium
and mivacurium. Doxacurium is the most potent agent available and has
no cardiovascular side effects. These drugs are used in anaesthesia.

Case 134

Q134.1 What is the diagnosis?

A134.1

Pulmonary hypertension with compression of the recurrent laryngeal
nerve by a dilated pulmonary artery. The mid-diastolic murmur may be
a right ventricular third heart sound. Mitral stenosis is unlikely, as the
first heart sound is soft. There is an association between schistosomiasis
and pulmonary hypertension.

Q134.2 What are the causes of this disorder?

A134.2

These are: idiopathic, ASD, recurrent PE, collagen diseases, sarcoidosis, mitral stenosis, chronic lung disease and alveolar hypoventilation.

Q134.3 How would you investigate her?

A134.3

One should perform a *V/Q* scan, echocardiography and pulmonary catheterisation with angiography. A lung function test should also be performed. A lung biopsy is rarely required; it is dangerous in the presence of raised pulmonary artery pressure.

Case 135

Q135.1 What is the diagnosis?

A135.1

De Quervain's thyroiditis. A viral aetiology has been implicated. The thyroid gland is usually diffusely tender.

Q135.2 How is it diagnosed?

A135.2

A radio-uptake scan will reveal almost absent uptake in the thyroid gland. The raised thyroid hormone level is due to the inflammatory destruction of the tissue. This is consistent with any form of thyroiditis.

Q135.3 How would you treat her?

A135.3

She should be given analgesics. Severe cases may require oral prednisolone. The majority of patients remain euthyroid but some may become permanently hypothyroid.

Supplementary Question Q135.4   How would you manage a thyroid crisis or storm?

Supplementary Answer A135.4

The classic presentation is that of fever and dysrhythmias, with hypotension and both neurological and gastrointestinal symptoms. The neurological manifestations include confusion and agitation, and the abdominal symptoms are pain and vomiting.

The management includes i.v. β-blockers, carbimazole and re-hydration. Atrial fibrillation may require digoxin and the patient should be adequately sedated. Some units use sodium iodide an hour after the first dose of carbimazole to prevent any further release of thyroxin from the gland. Blood should be sent for thyroid hormones and autoanti-bodies.